Fertility Diet

Cookbook For Women

:

Dietary Approach To Take Care Of Your Body And Getting Ready For Conception With Preconception Nutrition And Fertility Enlightenment.

Lee G. Johnson

Table Of Contents

About The Book

Fertility Diet Cookbook For Women : This is a comprehensive guide designed to support individuals and couples on their quest to conceive and build a family. Divided into two distinct parts, the book offers a balance of theoretical insights and practical advice to empower readers throughout their fertility journey.

Part I:

Theoretical Foundations : In the first part of the book, readers delve into the theoretical foundations of fertility, reproductive health, and the various factors that can influence conception. Chapters cover topics such as:

Understanding Fertility: Exploring the biological processes of conception, ovulation, and sperm production.

Hormonal Balance: Discussing the role of hormones in fertility and how imbalances can impact reproductive health.

Psychological Factors: Examining the emotional and psychological aspects of infertility, stress management, and coping strategies.

Lifestyle and Environmental Factors: Identifying lifestyle choices, environmental toxins, and dietary habits that may affect fertility.

Treatment Options: Providing an overview of fertility treatments, including assisted reproductive technologies (ART), medications, and alternative therapies.

Part II:

Practical Guidance and Recipes The second part of the book focuses on practical guidance and provides a collection of fertility-friendly recipes that incorporate nutrient-rich ingredients and culinary techniques to enhance fertility. Chapters include:

Nutrition and Diet: Offering dietary recommendations, fertility-boosting foods, and meal plans to support reproductive health.

Meal Planning for Fertility: Offering tips and strategies for meal planning, grocery shopping, and pantry stocking to support fertility goals.

Fertility-Boosting Breakfasts: Providing recipes for nourishing breakfast options such as smoothies, overnight oats, and nutrient-rich breakfast bowls.

Power-Packed Lunches: Featuring recipes for balanced and satisfying lunches that include salads, wraps, soups, and grain bowls filled with fertility-friendly ingredients.

Wholesome Dinners: Presenting a variety of dinner recipes that highlight lean proteins, whole grains, and colorful vegetables to create nutritious and delicious meals for fertility support.

Snacks and Treats: Offering ideas for fertility-friendly snacks and treats that provide energy and satisfy cravings while supporting reproductive health.

Special Occasions and Celebrations: Providing recipes for special occasions and celebrations, including festive meals and desserts that align with fertility nutrition principles.

A Guide to Cooking for Conception" serves as a comprehensive resource for individuals and couples seeking to optimize their fertility through nutrition and culinary creativity. By combining theoretical knowledge with practical recipes and cooking tips, this book empowers readers to take control of their fertility journey and nourish their bodies with delicious and wholesome meals designed to support conception and reproductive wellness.

This cookbook is designed to guide you through a delicious journey of foods that can support your fertility journey. Whether you're trying to conceive naturally or through assisted reproductive techniques, nourishing your body with wholesome, nutrient-rich foods can play a significant role in optimizing your fertility.

In this book, you'll find a variety of recipes crafted with ingredients known for their fertility-boosting properties. From vibrant salads to hearty main courses and delightful desserts, each recipe is thoughtfully curated to provide essential nutrients, support hormonal balance, and enhance overall well-being.

Remember, fertility is a holistic journey encompassing physical, emotional, and nutritional aspects. While this cookbook focuses on the nutritional component, it's essential to complement these recipes with a healthy lifestyle, stress management techniques, and, if needed, professional guidance from healthcare providers specializing in fertility.

Let's embark on this nourishing journey together and empower ourselves with the knowledge and flavors that support fertility and overall health.

Part One : Theoretical Approach

Chapter 1: Understanding Preconception Nutrition

- **Exploring the Importance of Preconception Nutrition**
- **Nutrients Essential for Fertility and Reproductive Health**
- **The Impact of Diet on Hormonal Balance**
- **Addressing Nutritional Deficiencies and Imbalances**

Exploring the Importance of Preconception Nutrition

Preparing for conception is an incredibly significant phase in a woman's life, one that involves a multitude of factors, including physical, emotional, and environmental considerations. Among these, nutrition plays a pivotal role in shaping fertility and laying the foundation for a healthy pregnancy.

Understanding the importance of preconception nutrition is the first step towards optimizing reproductive health and enhancing the chances of conception.

Nutrient Sufficiency: Preconception nutrition focuses on ensuring that the body is adequately nourished with essential vitamins, minerals, and macronutrients. These nutrients play vital roles in hormone regulation, reproductive function, and overall well-being. Deficiencies in key nutrients can impair fertility and increase the risk of complications during pregnancy.

Hormonal Balance: Hormonal balance is crucial for reproductive health and fertility. Certain nutrients, such as omega-3 fatty acids, zinc, and B vitamins, play key roles in hormone synthesis, regulation, and metabolism. A well-balanced diet can help maintain optimal hormonal levels, supporting menstrual regularity and ovulation.

Ovulation and Menstrual Health: Regular ovulation is essential for conception to occur. Nutritional factors, including body weight, insulin sensitivity, and micronutrient status, influence the menstrual cycle and ovulatory function. Maintaining a healthy weight through nutritious eating habits and lifestyle choices can help regulate menstrual cycles and improve fertility.

Optimizing Egg Quality: The quality of a woman's eggs is a critical determinant of fertility and pregnancy outcomes. Antioxidants, found abundantly in fruits, vegetables, and whole grains, help protect eggs from oxidative damage and preserve their integrity. Incorporating antioxidant-rich foods into the diet can enhance egg quality and reproductive potential.

Supporting Reproductive Organs: Nutrients such as folate, iron, and vitamin D are essential for the development and function of reproductive organs, including the ovaries and uterus. Adequate intake of these nutrients supports follicular development, implantation, and fetal growth during pregnancy.

Reducing Inflammation: Chronic inflammation has been linked to infertility and pregnancy complications. Certain dietary patterns, such as the Mediterranean diet, rich in anti-inflammatory foods like fatty fish, olive oil, and leafy greens, may help reduce inflammation and promote reproductive health.

Managing Weight and Metabolic Health: Maintaining a healthy weight and optimal metabolic health is important for fertility. Excess body weight can disrupt hormonal balance, impair ovulation, and increase the risk of conditions such as polycystic ovary syndrome (PCOS) and insulin resistance. A balanced diet, combined with regular physical activity, supports weight management and metabolic health.

In essence, preconception nutrition serves as a cornerstone for fertility and reproductive wellness. By nourishing the body with nutrient-dense foods, promoting hormonal balance, and supporting overall health, women can optimize their chances of conception and lay the groundwork for a healthy pregnancy and baby.

Nutrients Essential for Fertility and Reproductive Health

A careful balance of several nutrients that promote hormone control, egg quality, sperm health, and general reproductive function is necessary for optimal fertility and reproductive health. By including a wide variety of nutrient-dense foods in your diet, you may make sure that your body gets the fundamental components required for conception and pregnancy. The following are some vital nutrients needed for healthy reproduction and fertility:

Folate (Vitamin B9): This is necessary for early embryonic development and the prevention of neural tube abnormalities in developing fetuses because it plays a critical role in DNA synthesis and cell division. Citrus fruits, lentils, fortified grains, and leafy green vegetables are good sources of folate.

Iron: Iron is essential to the body's ability to carry oxygen, and it's especially critical for pregnant women to maintain appropriate blood hemoglobin levels. Lean meats, chicken, fish, beans, lentils, fortified cereals, and dark leafy greens are among the foods high in iron.

Omega-3 Fatty Acids: In particular, EPA (eicosapentaenoic acid) and DHA (docosahexaenoic acid) are essential for maintaining balanced hormone levels, lowering inflammation, and fostering the best possible quality in eggs and sperm. Walnuts, flaxseeds, chia seeds, salmon, mackerel, and sardines are good sources of omega-3 fatty acids, as are supplements made of algae.

Antioxidants: Antioxidants, which include zinc, selenium, vitamin C, and vitamin E, aid in preventing oxidative stress and damage from free radicals to reproductive cells. Berries, citrus fruits, nuts, seeds, green tea, and vibrantly colored veggies like spinach, bell peppers, and carrots are examples of foods high in antioxidants.

Iodine: Iodine is necessary for the creation of thyroid hormone, which is vital for controlling metabolism and promoting fertility. It's crucial for pregnant women to consume enough iodine in order to protect the developing baby. Seafood, dairy products, seaweed, and iodized salt are good sources of iodine.

Calcium and vitamin D: While vitamin D helps the body absorb calcium and maintains immune system function, calcium is essential for healthy bones and muscular function. Throughout pregnancy and nursing, these nutrients are essential for keeping strong bones and teeth. Leafy greens, fatty fish, dairy products, and fortified plant-based milk are food sources of calcium and vitamin D.

Zinc: Zinc is necessary for both male and female fertility as it is required for the manufacture of DNA, cell division, and hormone control. Pregnancy problems and infertility have been related to zinc deficiency. Lean meats, poultry, fish, nuts, seeds, whole grains, and legumes are foods that are good providers of zinc.

B vitamins: Vital for energy metabolism, neuron function, and DNA synthesis, B vitamins include B6, B12, and riboflavin (B2). These vitamins promote general reproductive health and have important functions in hormone control. Meat, fish, poultry, dairy products, eggs, leafy greens, and fortified cereals are among the foods that are good sources of B vitamins.

You may maximize your fertility and support your reproductive health by emphasizing nutrient-rich foods and keeping a balanced diet that includes a range of fruits, vegetables, whole grains, lean meats, and healthy fats. A healthy lifestyle that incorporates regular exercise, stress reduction methods, enough sleep, and abstaining from dangerous drugs like tobacco and excessive alcohol is crucial in addition to nutritional considerations.

The Impact of Diet on Hormonal Balance

Hormonal balance affects ovulation, regular menstruation, and overall fertility, making it a crucial component of reproductive health. Hormone levels are largely controlled by diet, as certain foods and nutrients may either support or interfere with hormonal balance. It is crucial to comprehend how nutrition affects hormonal balance in order to maximize fertility and promote reproductive health.

Blood Sugar Regulation with Insulin: Insulin may be released when blood sugar climbs due to diets high in refined carbs and sweets. Reduced sensitivity to insulin is the hallmark of insulin resistance, a disorder that may mess with hormone levels and ovulation. Consume complex carbs, foods high in fiber, and sources of healthy fats and proteins to help stabilize blood sugar levels and promote hormone balance.

Vitamin D Metabolism: One important reproductive hormone that is essential to both fertility and menstrual periods is estrogen. Estrogen is metabolized by the body by a number of processes, including hydroxylation and methylation. Some nutrients, such citrus fruits, flaxseeds, and cruciferous vegetables (broccoli, kale, Brussels sprouts), assist the liver's detoxification activities and help regulate estrogen levels. By including these items in your diet, you may lower your chance of developing estrogen dominance and encourage a healthy metabolism of estrogen.

Amino Acids and Proteins: The building blocks of protein, amino acids are necessary for the creation and control of hormones. Eating enough meals high in protein gives the body the amino acids it needs to make hormones including thyroid hormones, insulin, and reproductive hormones (like luteinizing hormone and follicle-stimulating hormone). For the sake of your general health and hormonal balance, include lean protein sources in your meals, such as quinoa, fish, chicken, and tofu.

Good Fats and Blood Pressure: For the synthesis of hormones and the integrity of cell membranes, healthy fats—such as omega-3 fatty acids and monounsaturated fats—are essential. Although it is often maligned in mainstream diets, cholesterol is a necessary precursor to steroid hormones including progesterone, estrogen, and testosterone. Hormone production and balance may be supported by including foods high in healthy fats, such as avocados, nuts, seeds, olive oil, fatty fish, and coconut oil, in your diet.

Co-factors and micronutrients: Vitamins and minerals are examples of micronutrients that function as co-factors in enzymatic activities that are involved in the production and metabolism of hormones. For instance, magnesium promotes insulin sensitivity and thyroid function, while vitamin B6 is required for the synthesis of neurotransmitters and steroid hormones. To promote hormonal balance and general well-being, make sure you consume enough micronutrient-rich foods, such as leafy greens, nuts, seeds, whole grains, and colorful fruits and vegetables.

Hydration and Cleansing: For detoxification and hormone function to be at their best, proper hydration is crucial. Consuming enough water supports the health of the liver and kidneys by assisting in the removal of pollutants and metabolic waste. Herbal drinks may help detoxification pathways and improve hormonal balance. Examples of these teas include dandelion root tea and green tea.

Reducing Stress and Intentional Eating: By raising cortisol levels and changing the way reproductive hormones are produced, long-term stress may throw off the balance of hormones. Reducing stress by engaging in activities like yoga, mindfulness, deep breathing, and meditation might lessen the impact of stress on hormone levels. Digestion and nutrition absorption may also be aided by developing mindful eating practices, such as enjoying each

meal and being aware of hunger and fullness
signals.

Addressing Nutritional Deficiencies and Imbalances

Infertility and reproductive health may be greatly impacted by nutritional deficiencies and imbalances, which can result in irregular menstrual cycles, hormone dysregulation, and decreased chances of conception. Optimizing fertility and promoting general well-being require identifying and treating these deficits. The following list of typical nutritional imbalances and deficiencies, along with treatment options, should be noted:

Iron Insufficiency: Anemia, which results in weariness, weakness, and poor oxygen delivery throughout the body, may be caused by an iron shortage. Iron deficiency may be more common in women who eat a vegetarian or vegan diet or who have excessive menstrual flow. Include iron-rich foods in your diet, such as lean meats, chicken, fish, beans, lentils, fortified cereals, and dark leafy greens, to treat iron deficiency. Iron absorption may be improved by eating meals high in iron together with foods high in vitamin C, such citrus fruits or bell peppers.

Deficiency in Folate and Vitamin B12: Vitamin B12 and folate (vitamin B9) are necessary for cell division, DNA synthesis, and brain function. Deficiencies in these vitamins may lead to infertility and raise the chance of neural tube abnormalities in the growing baby. Eat foods high in these nutrients, such as leafy greens, citrus fruits, fortified grains, lean meats, fish, eggs, and dairy products, to treat folate and vitamin B12 insufficiency. If the deficit continues, or if you are following a particular diet, you may want to think about supplementing.

An imbalance of omega-3 fatty acids: Reproductive problems, hormone abnormalities, and inflammation may all be attributed to an imbalance between omega-3 and omega-6 fatty acids. Although omega-6 fatty acids are necessary, an imbalance between the ratio of omega-3 to omega-6 results from the overconsumption of these fatty acids in contemporary diets. To help fertility and rebalance fatty acid levels, raise your diet of omega-3-rich foods including walnuts, flaxseeds, chia seeds, and fatty fish (salmon, mackerel, sardines), as well as algae-based supplements.

Deficiency of Vitamin D: In order to maintain healthy bones, the immune system, and hormone balance, vitamin D is essential. Vitamin D deficiency has been connected to irregular menstruation, infertility, and pregnancy difficulties. Elevate your sun exposure, eat foods high in vitamin D, including egg yolks, dairy products with added calcium, and fatty fish, and if your vitamin D levels are low, think about taking supplements.

Deficiency in Iodine: Thyroid hormone production, which affects metabolism and reproductive function, requires iodine. Thyroid problems and decreased fertility are two consequences of iodine deficiency. To make sure you're getting enough iodine, eat seaweed, dairy products, seafood, and iodized salt. See a doctor if you're worried about the health of your thyroid or iodine levels.

Insufficient Antioxidants: Antioxidants are essential for maintaining fertility and shielding reproductive cells from oxidative damage. Egg and sperm quality may be negatively impacted by deficiencies in antioxidants such zinc, vitamin C, vitamin E, and selenium. To correct deficits and maintain reproductive health, increase your consumption of foods high in antioxidants, such as berries, citrus fruits, nuts, seeds, green tea, and colorful vegetables.

Intake of Protein and Amino Acids: The creation of hormones, cell structure, and reproductive function all depend on protein and amino acids. Hormone balance and fertility might be negatively impacted by a diet low in protein. Make sure you are getting enough lean protein from foods like fish, chicken, tofu, lentils, and quinoa to support your general health and reproductive health.

Chapter 2: Building a Fertile Foundation: The Role of Diet and Lifestyle

- **Creating a Fertility-Friendly Diet**
- **Incorporating Whole Foods and Nutrient-Rich Ingredients**
- **The Importance of Hydration and Detoxification**
- **Managing Stress and Cultivating Emotional Well-Being**

Creating a Fertility-Friendly Diet

The process of creating a diet that promotes fertility entails choosing foods high in nutrients that assist hormone balance, reproductive health, and general wellbeing. A balanced diet helps maximize fertility and raise the chance of becoming pregnant. When designing an eating plan that supports fertility, keep the following important points in mind:

Emphasis on Whole Foods: Eat a diet high in whole, minimally processed foods including vegetables, fruits, whole grains, legumes, lean meats, and healthy fats. Essential nutrients, fiber, and phytonutrients included in whole diets promote health and fertility.

Include Foods Based on Plants: Plant-based foods including fruits, vegetables, nuts, seeds, beans, and legumes should be emphasized. Antioxidants, fiber, and phytonutrients included in plant-based diets have been shown to lower inflammation, promote hormone balance, and enhance reproductive health.

Put Protein First: Incorporate high-quality protein sources into your diet to promote healthy reproduction, hormone synthesis, and egg quality. Choose lean protein sources such Greek yogurt, tofu, tempeh, fish, chicken, and eggs. Protein should be a part of every meal and snack in order to keep blood sugar levels steady and encourage fullness.

Select Good Fats: Incorporate healthy fat sources into your diet to aid in the synthesis of hormones, lower inflammation, and improve the absorption of nutrients. Include foods high in omega-3 fatty acids (found in fatty fish, flaxseeds, chia seeds, walnuts), and monounsaturated fats (found in avocados, olive oil, nuts) in your meals and snacks.

Make Fiber-Rich Foods a Priority: Make sure to eat a lot of foods high in fiber, such as whole grains, legumes, seeds, fruits, and vegetables. In addition to promoting satiety and blood sugar regulation, fiber helps maintain intestinal health. Select whole grains over refined grains, such as barley, quinoa, brown rice, and oats.

Add Nutrients That Boost Fertility: Include foods high in minerals that may increase fertility, such as antioxidants, vitamin D, iron, zinc, selenium, and folate. Select a range of vibrant fruits and vegetables to optimize your intake of nutrients. Add iron-rich foods like beans, lentils, lean meats, and dark green vegetables. Eat foods high in zinc, such as chicken, shellfish, nuts, seeds, and whole grains.

Maintain Hydration: Stay hydrated and promote general health throughout the day by drinking plenty of water. Digestion, detoxification, and hormone balance all depend on getting enough water. Reduce your consumption of sugar-filled drinks and replace them with infused water, herbal teas, and water.

Cut Back on Added Sugars and Processed Foods: Reduce your intake of sugary snacks, drinks, and highly processed meals since they might aggravate insulin resistance, inflammation, and hormone abnormalities. When it comes to eating, try to stick to whole, nutrient-dense meals and avoid items with artificial additives and added sweets.

Moderate Use of Alcohol and Caffeine: Limit your intake of alcohol and caffeine since these substances may have a deleterious effect on hormone balance and fertility. Choose decaffeinated drinks, herbal teas, and moderation when it comes to occasional indulgences.

Engage in Mindful Eating: Savor each mouthful of your meal and pay attention to its aromas and textures as you eat mindfully, paying attention to your body's signals of hunger and fullness. In addition to supporting digestion and enhancing general wellbeing, mindful eating may assist avoid overindulging.

Incorporating Whole Foods and Nutrient-Rich Ingredients

Incorporating whole foods and nutrient-rich items that provide vital vitamins, minerals, antioxidants, and phytonutrients required for hormonal balance and reproductive health is the first step in creating a diet that supports fertility. The following are doable methods for include these items in your regular meals:

Vibrantly colored fruits and veggies: As a rainbow of vibrant fruits and veggies that are high in antioxidants, fiber, vitamins, and minerals, pile them onto your plate. Add colorful veggies such as bell peppers, carrots, tomatoes, and beets, along with leafy greens like spinach, kale, and Swiss chard. To enhance general health and optimize nutritional intake, try to eat a rainbow of colors.

Complete Grains: Select whole grains instead of refined grains, such as bulgur, farro, quinoa, brown rice, and oats. Minerals including iron, magnesium, and selenium, as well as fiber and B vitamins, are abundant in whole grains. For increased nutrition and fullness, try adding whole grains to salads, stir-fries, soups, and grain bowls.

Trim Proteins: To maintain the health of your muscles, hormone production, and reproductive system, include sources of lean protein in your diet. Choose lean chicken, fish, seafood, tofu, tempeh, lentils, and bean products. To add diversity to your meals, try experimenting with plant-based protein sources like quinoa, edamame, chickpeas, and beans.

Good Fats: To promote hormone balance, cognitive function, and nutritional absorption, include sources of healthy fats in your diet. Select meals high in omega-3 fatty acids and monounsaturated fats, such as walnuts, flaxseeds, chia seeds, avocados, and olive oil. To add extra nutrition to salads and sandwiches, slice avocados, spread olive oil over roasted veggies, and add nuts and seeds to oatmeal or yogurt.

Dairy and its Substitutes: To promote bone health and supply calcium, vitamin D, and protein, include dairy products like yogurt, kefir, and cheese in your diet, or substitute dairy products with almond milk, soy milk, and coconut yogurt. To reduce additional sugars, choose for unsweetened types; add taste and extra nutrients by adding fresh fruit, nuts, and seeds.

Nut butters, seeds, and nuts: Add some healthy fats, protein, fiber, and micronutrients to your meals and snacks by including nuts, seeds, and nut butters. For extra nutrition, add ground flaxseeds or chia seeds to smoothies, cereal, or yogurt. You can also put nut butter over whole grain bread or fruit slices. Snackle on a handful of almonds, walnuts, or pumpkin seeds.

Spices and Herbs: Use herbs and spices like turmeric, ginger, garlic, cinnamon, and oregano to improve the taste and nutritional content of your food. In addition to giving meals depth and variety, herbs and spices include strong anti-inflammatory and antioxidant properties that promote general health and wellbeing.

Plant-Based Proteins: Try including more plant-based protein sources into your diet, such as seitan, tofu, tempeh, beans, lentils, and chickpeas, to help you feel less dependent on animal products. Rich in fiber, vitamins, minerals, and phytonutrients, plant-based proteins have been shown to support reproductive health and general well-being.

Prepared Dinners and Snacks: Make homemade meals and snacks a priority whenever you can, using whole, minimally processed products. Use seasonal, fresh ingredients to make homemade meals as often as possible; avoid relying too much on boxed and convenience foods. To make meal preparation and planning easier, batch cook grains, beans, and proteins in advance.

Drinking plenty of water: Make sure you drink plenty of water, herbal teas, and infused water to stay hydrated throughout the day. Maintaining proper digestion, vitamin absorption, detoxification, and general health all depend on enough hydration. To keep hydrated and alert, always have a reusable water bottle with you and take frequent sip of liquids.

The Importance of Hydration and Detoxification

Hydration and detoxification are essential processes that support overall health, including reproductive health and fertility. Proper hydration and effective detoxification mechanisms help maintain optimal physiological function, eliminate toxins, and support the body's natural ability to conceive and sustain a healthy pregnancy. Here's why hydration and detoxification are crucial for fertility:

Hydration for Reproductive Health: Adequate hydration is essential for reproductive health and fertility. Water plays a crucial role in maintaining the body's fluid balance, regulating body temperature, supporting nutrient transport, and facilitating waste removal. Proper hydration helps ensure optimal blood flow to reproductive organs, including the ovaries and uterus, which is essential for hormone production, egg quality, and uterine lining thickness.

Cervical Mucus Production: Proper hydration is necessary for the production of cervical mucus, which plays a critical role in fertility and conception. Cervical mucus serves as a medium for sperm transport, provides nourishment and protection to sperm cells, and helps facilitate their journey through the female reproductive tract. Inadequate hydration can lead to reduced cervical mucus production and impaired sperm transport, potentially hindering conception.

Detoxification Pathways: The body's detoxification pathways, primarily involving the liver, kidneys, lymphatic system, and digestive system, play a crucial role in eliminating metabolic waste products, environmental toxins, and excess hormones from the body. Proper hydration supports detoxification by promoting kidney function, facilitating the elimination of waste products through urine, and maintaining optimal liver function.

Elimination of Environmental Toxins: Exposure to environmental toxins, such as heavy metals, pesticides, endocrine-disrupting chemicals, and pollutants, can interfere with hormone balance, impair reproductive function, and increase the risk of infertility and pregnancy complications. Adequate hydration supports the elimination of toxins through urine and sweat, reducing the body's toxic burden and supporting reproductive health.

Optimal Egg and Sperm Quality: Hydration plays a role in maintaining optimal egg and sperm quality, which are crucial factors in fertility and conception. Proper hydration helps support cellular function, DNA integrity, and mitochondrial health, all of which contribute to healthy egg and sperm development. Dehydration can lead to cellular stress, oxidative damage, and compromised reproductive function.

Uterine Lining Thickness: Hydration is essential for maintaining adequate uterine lining thickness, which is necessary for embryo implantation and pregnancy establishment.

Proper hydration supports uterine blood flow and tissue hydration, ensuring an optimal environment for embryo implantation and early fetal development.

Reduced Risk of Ovulatory Dysfunction: Chronic dehydration may increase the risk of ovulatory dysfunction and menstrual irregularities, leading to infertility or subfertility. Proper hydration supports hormonal balance, ovarian function, and menstrual cycle regularity, optimizing the chances of conception.

**To promote hydration and support detoxification for optimal fertility, consider the following tips:**

- Drink plenty of water throughout the day, aiming for at least 8-10 glasses of water daily, or more if you're physically active or in hot weather.

- Incorporate hydrating foods such as water-rich fruits and vegetables (e.g., cucumber, watermelon, oranges, strawberries, lettuce) into your meals and snacks.

- Limit consumption of dehydrating beverages such as caffeinated drinks, alcohol, and sugary sodas, which can contribute to dehydration.

- Support detoxification by consuming a nutrient-rich diet that includes plenty of fruits, vegetables, whole grains, lean proteins, and healthy fats.

- Practice healthy lifestyle habits such as regular physical activity, stress management techniques, adequate sleep, and avoidance of environmental toxins to support overall health and fertility.

Managing Stress and Cultivating Emotional Well-Being

The cultivation of emotional well-being and stress management are essential components of reproductive health and fertility. Long-term stress may have a deleterious effect on menstrual cycles, fertility, and hormone balance; on the other hand, mental wellness is crucial for resilience and general health. The following are methods to reduce stress and promote mental health in order to aid in fertility:

Meditation & Mindfulness: Engage in mindfulness meditation to develop relaxation, lower stress levels, and a more present-moment awareness. By practicing mindfulness, one may reduce worry, calm the mind, and strengthen emotional fortitude. Every day, set aside some time to practice meditation. During this time, pay attention to your breath, your body, or a guided meditation.

The Mind-Body Connection with Yoga: Take part in mild yoga exercises that put an emphasis on stress relief, deep breathing, and relaxation. Yoga eases physical stress, soothes the neurological system, and improves awareness of the mind and body. To support emotional equilibrium and wellbeing, include gentle stretches, relaxation methods, and restorative yoga positions into your practice.

Breathing Techniques: To induce the relaxation response and lower stress levels, engage in deep breathing techniques like diaphragmatic breathing, box breathing, or alternate nostril breathing. Deep breathing exercises aid in mental calmness, emotional control, and the development of a sense of serenity and center.

Writing with Expression and Journaling: Expressive writing and journaling are great ways to explore your ideas, feelings, and experiences. You may develop self-awareness, understand your feelings, and process emotions via writing. Allocate a certain period of time every day for writing openly about your ideas, dreams, worries, and goals around conception and reproduction.

Social Links and Support: Seek out the understanding, empathy, and encouragement of loved ones, friends, support groups, or mental health experts. It is possible to reduce feelings of loneliness, normalize your emotions, and create a sense of connection and belonging by talking to people about your experiences and feelings.

Establishing Limits and Making Self-Care a Priority: Prioritize self-care activities that feed your body, mind, and soul, and set up appropriate boundaries to safeguard your emotional wellbeing. Assign work when it's necessary, set reasonable goals for yourself, and respect your desire for downtime, renewal, and leisure.

Developing Positivity and Gratitude: Consider the benefits and richness in your life to help you cultivate an attitude of thankfulness and optimism. Maintain a thankfulness diary where you may record happy, beautiful, and appreciative experiences from each day. Adopt a hopeful and upbeat mindset and have faith in the process of conception and reproduction.

Looking for Expert Assistance: See a therapist, counselor, or mental health expert for professional help if overwhelming emotions of stress, anxiety, or depression occur. They may provide advice, coping mechanisms, and therapeutic treatments customized to your needs.

Taking Part in Happy and Creative Activities: Take part in enjoyable and creative pursuits that make you feel happy, fulfilled, and purposeful. Investigate interests, loves, and pastimes that feed your spirit, spark your creativity, and provide a constructive way to express yourself and decompress.

Applying Forgiveness and Self-Compassion: As you manage the difficulties of conception and fertility, treat yourself with kindness and care. Treating oneself with love, understanding, and acceptance is a great way to practice self-compassion. Develop an attitude of forgiveness and let go of blame, anger, and self-judgment.

Chapter 3: Optimizing Fertility Through Nutrient-Rich Foods

- **Powerhouse Foods for Fertility Enhancement**
- **Understanding the Role of Macronutrients and Micronutrients**
- **Incorporating Antioxidants and Phytonutrients into Your Diet**
- **Superfoods for Super Fertility: A Comprehensive Guide**

Powerhouse Foods for Fertility Enhancement

Reproductive health and fertility are significantly influenced by nutrition. Your chances of becoming pregnant can be raised, egg and sperm quality can be optimized, and hormone balance can be supported by eating a diet rich in nutrients. The following foods are superfoods that you should include in your diet to increase fertility:

Greens with leaves: Rich in iron, antioxidants, and folate are leafy greens like spinach, kale, and Swiss chard. Folate lowers the chance of neural tube abnormalities in the developing baby and promotes good egg development. Iron promotes healthy blood flow to the reproductive organs and aids in the prevention of anemia.

Berries: Blackberries, raspberries, strawberries, and blueberries are rich in polyphenols and vitamin C, two types of antioxidants. Antioxidants increase general fertility by shielding reproductive cells from oxidative damage.

Saturated Fish: Omega-3 fatty acids, EPA, and DHA are abundant in salmon, mackerel, sardines, and trout. Reduced inflammation, improved sperm and egg quality, and boost hormone synthesis are all benefits of omega-3 fatty acids.

Avocado: Avocados are high in potassium, folate, vitamin E, and monounsaturated fats. Vitamin E functions as an antioxidant, shielding reproductive cells from harm, while monounsaturated fats promote hormone balance and reproductive health.

Seeds and Nuts: Rich in protein, fiber, good fats, and minerals include almonds, walnuts, flaxseeds, chia seeds, and pumpkin seeds. They provide vital minerals that help fertilization and reproductive function, such zinc, selenium, omega-3 fatty acids, and vitamin E.

Legumes: Iron, fiber, folate, and plant-based protein may be found in abundance in beans, lentils, chickpeas, and peas. They provide vital nutrients for reproductive health, maintain hormone balance, and control blood sugar.

Complete Grains: Rich in fiber, B vitamins, and minerals like selenium and magnesium are whole grains like quinoa, brown rice, oats, barley, and buckwheat. B vitamins promote hormone synthesis and energy metabolism, while fiber helps control hormone levels and enhances insulin sensitivity.

Eggs: Rich in protein, choline, and vitamin D, eggs are a nutrient-dense food that supports healthy reproduction and fertility. While vitamin D controls hormone levels and boosts the immune system, choline aids in the development of the fetus's brain.

Greek yogurt: Probiotics, calcium, and protein are all abundant in Greek yogurt. Calcium is necessary for healthy bones and muscular function, while protein promotes hormone production and egg quality. Probiotics may assist reproductive health and gastrointestinal health.

Bright Vegetables: Rich in vitamins, minerals, and antioxidants include bell peppers, carrots, tomatoes, and sweet potatoes. Vegetables that are orange or yellow include beta-carotene, which promotes reproductive health and may increase fertility.

Understanding the Role of Macronutrients and Micronutrients

Fertility is greatly impacted by nutrition, which also affects hormone balance, reproductive health, and general well-being. Both macronutrients and micronutrients are necessary for a balanced diet that promotes the highest possible level of fertility. Making educated food decisions to increase your chances of conception may be aided by your understanding of their responsibilities. An outline of the roles played by macro and micronutrients in fertility is provided below:

Macronutrients

Glucose: The body uses carbohydrates as its main energy source and needs them to sustain hormone synthesis and metabolic processes. Choose complex carbs over simple ones. Whole grains, fruits, vegetables, and legumes are good sources of nutrients and long-lasting energy that also help to control blood sugar levels.

Proteins: As the building blocks of life, proteins are essential for the production of hormones, the development of eggs and sperm, and the operation of the reproductive system. Sufficient consumption of protein promotes sperm production, ovulation, and embryo implantation. Incorporate into your diet lean protein sources including fish, chicken, eggs, dairy, tofu, tempeh, lentils, and nuts.

Lipids: Reproductive health, cell membrane integrity, and hormone synthesis all depend on healthy fats. Fatty fish, flaxseeds, chia seeds, walnuts, and algae-based supplements are good sources of omega-3 fatty acids, which are beneficial for developing embryos, sperm motility, and egg quality. Consume monounsaturated fats to enhance reproductive health and hormone balance, such as those found in almonds, avocados, and olive oil.

Micronutrients

Folate, or vitamin B9: Folate is necessary for the fetus's neural tube development, cell division, and DNA synthesis. Sufficient consumption of folate promotes early embryonic development and lowers the chance of neural tube abnormalities. Citrus fruits, lentils, fortified grains, and leafy green vegetables are good sources of folate.

Iron: Red blood cell creation, energy generation, and oxygen delivery all need iron. Anemia from iron deficiency may affect fertility and raise the possibility of pregnancy problems. Eat foods high in iron, such as fish, poultry, beans, lentils, lean meats, fortified cereals, and dark green vegetables.

Zinc: Zinc is necessary for fertility and reproductive health because it plays a role in hormone control, DNA synthesis, and cell division. A zinc deficit may affect the development of embryos, ovulation, and sperm production. Consume foods high in zinc, such as legumes, whole grains, nuts, seeds, poultry, fish, and lean meats.

Vitamin D: Immune system performance, calcium absorption, and hormone control all depend heavily on vitamin D. Pregnancy problems, irregular menstruation, and infertility have all been related to vitamin D insufficiency. Sunlight exposure, fatty fish, fortified dairy products, and supplements, if necessary, are good sources of vitamin D.

Vitamins C, E, and selenium are antioxidants: Antioxidants aid in defending reproductive cells from free radical-induced oxidative damage. Selenium, vitamin C, and vitamin E promote the health of sperm, the quality of eggs, and reproductive processes. Consume foods high in antioxidants, such as seafood, nuts, seeds, citrus fruits, berries, and green leafy vegetables.

Iodine: Thyroid hormone production, which controls metabolism and promotes reproductive health, requires iodine. Thyroid problems and decreased fertility are two consequences of iodine deficiency. To make sure you're getting enough iodine, eat seaweed, dairy products, seafood, and iodized salt.

B vitamins: riboflavin, B6, and B12: Hormone production, energy metabolism, and neural tube development are all impacted by B vitamins. Sufficient consumption of B vitamins promotes hormone homeostasis, fertility, and successful pregnancy outcomes. Meat, fish, poultry, dairy products, eggs, leafy greens, and fortified cereals are some examples of sources.

Incorporating Antioxidants and Phytonutrients into Your Diet

Strong substances called phytonutrients and antioxidants are included in plant-based diets and are essential for promoting hormone balance, preventing oxidative damage to reproductive cells, and increasing fertility. Including a range of foods high in phytonutrients and antioxidants in your diet may help to support reproductive health and improve your chances of becoming pregnant. Here's how to improve fertility by include antioxidants and phytonutrients in your diet:

Vibrantly colored fruits and veggies: Include as many different hues of fruits and vegetables as possible in your meals and snacks. Select kinds with intense pigmentation, such purple cabbage, kale, spinach, oranges, kiwis, and mangoes. Antioxidants such as vitamin C, vitamin E, beta-carotene, and flavonoids are abundant in these colorful meals and help shield reproductive cells from oxidative stress while promoting fertility.

Berries: Antioxidants, including anthocyanins and polyphenols, are abundant in berries, including blueberries, strawberries, raspberries, and blackberries. These compounds have anti-inflammatory and protective properties for reproductive health. Fresh berries may be eaten as a cool snack or added to smoothies, yogurt, cereal, and salads.

Greens with leaves: Rich in antioxidants, vitamins, and minerals that are necessary for fertility, leafy green vegetables including spinach, kale, Swiss chard, and collard greens are a great source of these nutrients. Folate, vitamin C, vitamin E, and lutein are found in these greens, and they boost reproductive health, hormone balance, and egg quality. Add leafy greens to omelets, stir-fries, soups, salads, and green smoothies.

Cruciferous Squash: Sulfur compounds and phytonutrients including glucosinolates, indole-3-carbinol, and sulforaphane are found in cruciferous vegetables like broccoli, cauliflower, Brussels sprouts, and cabbage. These chemicals assist hormone metabolism, detoxification pathways, and reproductive health. Cruciferous vegetables may be added to stir-fries, salads, or roasted or steamed as a side dish.

Vibrant Peppers: Flavonoids, beta-carotene, and vitamin C are among the many antioxidants found in bell peppers, particularly the red, yellow, and orange types. These antioxidants assist in reducing inflammation, counteracting free radical damage, and protecting reproductive cells from oxidative harm. Sliced bell peppers are great as a crisp snack, added to salads, or used in fajitas and stir-fries.

Tomatoes: Lycopene, an antioxidant linked to better sperm quality and a lower risk of male infertility, is abundant in tomatoes. Higher amounts of lycopene may be found in cooked and processed tomatoes, such as those used to make salsa, tomato paste, and sauce. Add tomatoes to salads, sandwiches, soups, and sauces to increase their antioxidant content.

Seeds and Nuts: Nuts and seeds are full of vitamins, minerals, protein, fiber, and healthy fats. Some examples of nuts and seeds include walnuts, almonds, flaxseeds, chia seeds, and pumpkin seeds. Additionally, they include antioxidants that help hormone balance and reproductive health, such vitamin E, selenium, and lignans. Nuts and seeds may be added to yogurt, salads, cereal, or eaten as a high-nutrient snack.

Spices and Herbs: Add spices and herbs to your food, such as garlic, oregano, ginger, turmeric, and cinnamon. These tasty additions offer anti-inflammatory and immune-stimulating qualities since they are high in antioxidants, polyphenols, and phytonutrients. For more taste and nutritional advantages, season foods, marinades, sauces, and dressings with herbs and spices.

Green Tea: Strong antioxidants called catechins, which are found in green tea, have been linked to better reproductive results in both men and women. Drink green tea as a cool drink or blend it into smoothies and iced teas.

Dark Chocolate: Strong antioxidants called flavonoids, which are found in dark chocolate, may help cardiovascular health and enhance blood flow to the reproductive organs. As a rare treat, savor a little piece of dark chocolate with at least 70% cacao.

Superfoods for Super Fertility: A Comprehensive Guide

Unlocking the potential of superfoods can significantly enhance fertility and reproductive health. These nutrient-dense foods are rich in vitamins, minerals, antioxidants, and phytonutrients, offering a powerful boost to your fertility journey. Let's explore a comprehensive guide to superfoods for super fertility:

1. **Berries:** Blueberries, strawberries, raspberries, and blackberries are loaded with antioxidants, including vitamin C and flavonoids. These compounds help protect reproductive cells from oxidative damage, support hormone balance, and improve overall fertility.

2. **Leafy Greens:** Spinach, kale, Swiss chard, and collard greens are nutritional powerhouses packed with folate, iron, calcium, and vitamin K. These leafy greens support hormone regulation, promote healthy ovulation, and provide essential nutrients for fetal development.

3. Avocado: Avocado is a rich source of monounsaturated fats, vitamin E, potassium, and folate. These nutrients support hormone synthesis, egg quality, and reproductive health. Incorporate avocado into salads, smoothies, or as a creamy spread on toast.

4. Fatty Fish: Salmon, mackerel, sardines, and trout are abundant sources of omega-3 fatty acids, EPA, and DHA. These essential fats support hormone production, reduce inflammation, and enhance sperm and egg quality, improving fertility outcomes.

5. Nuts and Seeds: Almonds, walnuts, flaxseeds, chia seeds, and pumpkin seeds are packed with healthy fats, protein, fiber, and micronutrients. These superfoods support hormone balance, reproductive function, and sperm health, making them essential additions to a fertility-friendly diet.

6. Beans and Legumes: Beans, lentils, chickpeas, and peas are rich in protein, fiber, folate, and iron. These plant-based superfoods support menstrual regularity, hormone metabolism, and reproductive health. Incorporate beans and legumes into soups, stews, salads, and grain bowls for a nutrient boost.

7. Greek Yogurt: Greek yogurt is a protein-rich dairy option that provides calcium, probiotics, and vitamin D. Calcium supports uterine health and muscle function, while probiotics promote gut health and immune function, enhancing overall fertility.

8. Eggs: Eggs are a complete protein source rich in choline, vitamin D, and B vitamins. Choline supports fetal brain development, while vitamin D regulates hormone levels and supports reproductive health. Include eggs in your diet as a versatile and nutrient-dense option.

9. Quinoa: Quinoa is a gluten-free whole grain rich in protein, fiber, iron, and magnesium. These nutrients support hormone balance, blood sugar regulation, and reproductive function. Use quinoa as a nutritious base for salads, stir-fries, and grain bowls.

10. Turmeric: - Turmeric contains curcumin, a potent antioxidant and anti-inflammatory compound. Curcumin helps reduce inflammation, support immune function, and improve reproductive health. Incorporate turmeric into curries, soups, smoothies, or turmeric latte for its health benefits.

11. Dark Chocolate: - Dark chocolate with at least 70% cocoa content is rich in flavonoids and antioxidants. Enjoying a small piece of dark chocolate as an occasional treat can support cardiovascular health, reduce stress, and enhance fertility.

12. Maca Root: - Maca root is an adaptogenic herb known for its fertility-enhancing properties.

It supports hormone balance, libido, and reproductive function in both men and women. Add maca powder to smoothies, oatmeal, or energy balls for a natural fertility boost.

Chapter 4: Enhancing Fertility Through Mind-Body Connection

- **Exploring the Mind-Body Connection in Fertility**
- **Practicing Mindfulness and Stress Reduction Techniques**
- **Yoga, Meditation, and Breathing Exercises for Fertility**
- **Cultivating Positive Thoughts and Beliefs**

Exploring the Mind-Body Connection in Fertility

The process of fertility is not only physical; the mind-body link has a significant impact on it. The significance of treating mental and emotional aspects in fertility is shown by the interaction between stress levels, emotional well-being, and reproductive health. An examination of the mind-body link in fertility is provided below:

Stress and the Hormone System: Persistent stress may throw off the hormone balance, which can have an impact on menstrual cycles and the hypothalamic-pituitary-ovarian axis. Increased stress may cause irregular menstruation, irregular ovulation, and decreased fertility. Stress management practices including mindfulness, relaxation, and stress-reduction tactics may assist reestablish hormonal balance and enhance the success of conception.

Fertility and Emotional Health: Fertility and conception are significantly influenced by emotional health. Hormone levels, menstrual periods, and reproductive function may all be impacted by feelings of worry, melancholy, or unresolved emotional difficulties. Reproductive health and fertility may be favorably impacted by developing emotional resilience, asking for help from loved ones, and resolving emotional issues via treatment or counseling.

The Effects of Negative Thoughts and Beliefs: Fertility difficulties may be made worse by negative ideas and attitudes about conception, parenting, and fertility. These ideas and beliefs can lead to worry and anxiety. Rethinking ideas, challenging unfavorable views, and developing an optimistic outlook may all aid in lowering stress and fostering an atmosphere that is conducive to conception.

Techniques for Relaxation and Mindfulness: Deep breathing exercises, yoga, mindfulness meditation, and visualization methods are examples of mind-body activities that may help lower stress, increase relaxation, and improve fertility. These techniques support fertility by lowering cortisol levels, promoting a calm and balanced state of mind, and stimulating the body's relaxation response.

The Support Systems' Function: The presence of social support, community, and connection is essential for both mental and reproductive health. Having a solid support system of friends, family, online forums, and support groups may be a great way to get understanding, validation, and encouragement while going through the reproductive process. Speaking with people about your struggles, thoughts, and experiences may help you feel less alone and provide a lot of emotional support.

Comprehensive Methods for Fertility: In order to achieve optimum reproductive health, holistic approaches to fertility acknowledge the interdependence of the mind, body, and spirit. By treating underlying imbalances and enhancing general well-being, integrative therapies including acupuncture, chiropractic care, massage therapy, and naturopathic medicine may support traditional reproductive treatments.

Self-Care Routines and the Fertility Mindset: Having a proactive, empowered attitude to fertility and placing a high value on self-care routines that feed the mind, body, and spirit are all part of cultivating a fertility mentality.

Fertility may be improved and emotional well-being supported by partaking in joyful, fulfilling, and relaxing activities including hobbies, artistic endeavors, nature walks, and self-care routines.

Communication and Support amongst Couples: The marriage connection must have effective communication and mutual support in order to overcome the obstacles of infertility and fertility therapy. In order to build resilience in the face of shared reproductive challenges, couples should strengthen their link via open and honest communication, empathy, and shared decision-making.

<u>**Practicing Mindfulness and Stress Reduction Techniques**</u>

Your fertility journey may be significantly impacted by including stress-reduction and mindfulness practices into your everyday routine. Through the practice of awareness cultivation, stress management, and emotional well-being promotion, you may establish an internal environment that is supportive to conception. Consider the following mindfulness and stress-reduction methods:

Methods for Mindful Breathing: To ease tension and encourage relaxation, try deep breathing techniques. Locate a peaceful area, get into a comfortable position, and inhale deeply and slowly. Allow your mind to settle into a state of quiet center while you concentrate on the feeling of the breath coming into and going out of your body.

Meditation with the body scan: Try a body scan meditation to help you relax and relieve stress all throughout your body. Raising awareness of each portion of your body, begin with your toes and work your way up gradually. Breathe deeply, noticing any places of tension or pain, and releasing them gently.

Walking With Awareness: To de-stress and establish a connection with the present, go for mindful walks in the outdoors. While you walk, pay attention to the sights, sounds, and feelings around you. Inhale the clean air, take in the hues of the sky and trees, and feel the earth under your feet.

Directed Visualization and Imagery: To generate uplifting mental pictures associated with conception and fertility, engage in guided imagery and visualization practices. Shut your eyes, picture yourself in a calm, productive setting, and see your reproductive organs operating at full capacity. Give yourself permission to be at ease, hopeful, and optimistic.

Consciously Consuming Food: Savor every mouthful of your meals and pay attention to the aromas, textures, and feelings of the food as you engage in mindful eating. Chew your meal gently, take in its flavors and colors, and be grateful for the nutrients it gives your body.

Tai Chi and Yoga: Take up mild movement exercises like Tai Chi or yoga to increase your flexibility, awareness of your body, and ability to relax. These techniques, which include breathing exercises, meditation, and mild physical activity, might enhance general wellbeing by lowering stress and promoting better circulation.

Progressive Relaxation of the Muscles: Tensing and relaxing various muscle groups in your body in a methodical manner is the practice of progressive muscle relaxation. Tension each muscle group for a short while before letting go, starting with your toes and working your way up to your head. As you go through the procedure, take note of the tension and relaxation you experience.

Reflection and Journaling: Spend some time in your notebook thinking back on your conception-related events, emotions, and ideas. Jot down your dreams, worries, and goals together with any difficulties or barriers you may be encountering. Writing about yourself might help you get insight on your reproductive journey and let go of bottled up feelings.

Establishing Limits and Making Self-Care a Priority: Establish limits on your time, resources, and obligations so that you may give your mental health and self-care first priority. Saying no to commitments or activities that sap your energy and cause stress is a skill. Allocate time for pursuits that uplift and delight you.

Looking for Assistance and Relationships: During your path toward fertility, reach out to friends, family, support groups, or mental health experts for connection and support. Finding support, encouragement, and a sense of community may come from confiding in others who can relate to your experiences, feelings, and worries.

Yoga, Meditation, and Breathing Exercises for Fertility

Integrating yoga, meditation, and breathing exercises into your daily routine can offer profound benefits for fertility by reducing stress, promoting relaxation, and enhancing mind-body connection. These practices help create a supportive internal environment conducive to reproductive health and well-being. Here's how to incorporate yoga, meditation, and breathing exercises into your fertility journey:

Yoga Asanas for Fertility: Certain yoga poses can help improve circulation to the reproductive organs, balance hormone levels, and reduce stress. Consider incorporating the following yoga asanas into your practice:

- **Supta Baddha Konasana (Reclining Bound Angle Pose):** Opens the hips and pelvis, promoting blood flow to the reproductive organs.

- **Viparita Karani (Legs-Up-the-Wall Pose):** Improves circulation to the pelvic area and reduces stress.

- **Bharadvajasana (Bharadvaja's Twist):** Releases tension in the spine and stimulates digestion, supporting reproductive health.

- **Balasana (Child's Pose):** Calms the mind, relieves tension in the back and shoulders, and promotes relaxation.

Meditation for Fertility: Meditation is a powerful tool for reducing stress, calming the mind, and enhancing emotional well-being during the fertility journey. Consider practicing mindfulness meditation, focused meditation, or loving-kindness meditation to cultivate inner peace and resilience. Set aside time each day to sit quietly, focus on your breath, and observe your thoughts and emotions without judgment.

Breathing Exercises for Fertility: Deep breathing exercises can help activate the body's relaxation response, reduce stress hormones, and promote optimal oxygenation to the reproductive organs. Practice the following breathing techniques regularly:

1. **Deep Belly Breathing:** Sit or lie down comfortably, place one hand on your abdomen, and inhale deeply through your nose, allowing your belly to expand. Exhale slowly through your mouth, feeling your belly deflate. Repeat for several breaths, focusing on the rhythm of your breath.

2. **Alternate Nostril Breathing (Nadi Shodhana):** Sit in a comfortable position, use your right thumb to close your right nostril, and inhale deeply through your left nostril. Close your left nostril with your ring finger, exhale through your right nostril, then inhale through your right nostril. Close your right nostril, exhale

through your left nostril, and continue alternating for several breaths.

3. **4-7-8 Breathing:** Inhale deeply through your nose for a count of four, hold your breath for a count of seven, then exhale slowly through your mouth for a count of eight. Repeat this cycle several times, allowing yourself to relax and release tension with each exhale.

Yoga Nidra for Fertility: Yoga Nidra, or yogic sleep, is a guided relaxation technique that promotes deep relaxation and rejuvenation. Lie down in a comfortable position, close your eyes, and follow a guided Yoga Nidra practice to release physical tension, calm the mind, and restore balance to the body. Yoga Nidra can help reduce stress, improve sleep quality, and enhance overall well-being during the fertility journey.

Fertility-Focused Yoga and Meditation Classes: Consider attending fertility-focused yoga and meditation classes or workshops led by experienced instructors who understand the unique needs of individuals on their fertility journey. These specialized classes may incorporate gentle yoga sequences, meditation practices, and breathing exercises specifically designed to support reproductive health and emotional well-being.

Consistency and Commitment: Establish a regular yoga, meditation, and breathing practice that fits your schedule and preferences. Set aside dedicated time each day to nourish your body, mind, and spirit through these transformative practices. Consistency and commitment to your practice will help you reap the full benefits of yoga, meditation, and breathing exercises for fertility.

Cultivating Positive Thoughts and Beliefs

Your road towards fertility may be significantly impacted by the power of good thoughts and attitudes. Reducing stress, improving mental health, and creating an atmosphere inside that is favorable to conception are all possible via positive attitude cultivation. The following are some methods to foster constructive ideas and conceptions for fertility:

Exercise Gratitude: Consider the things you have in your life for which you are grateful as you develop a daily practice of thankfulness. Every day, no matter how little, set aside some time to recognize and be grateful for the benefits, pleasures, and beautiful moments that surround you. By expressing your thankfulness, you may change your attention from what is missing to what is plentiful, which will increase your feeling of happiness and optimism.

Gratitude and constructive self-talk: Reframe negative attitudes and beliefs about fertility by including self-talk and positive affirmations into your everyday practice. Make affirmations that express your aspirations for conception and family and that speak to you personally. Regularly repeat these affirmations either loud or quietly to strengthen your positive thoughts and develop a resilient, hopeful, and self-assured mentality.

Envision the result you want: Use visualization exercises to see yourself feeling the happiness and contentment that come with becoming a parent. Shut your eyes and see yourself in the future holding your child and experiencing a profound sensation of love and connection. As you see your ideal result materializing, let yourself get fully enveloped in the emotions of happiness, appreciation, and expectation.

Concentrate on the Here and Now: To develop acceptance and serenity with where you are on your fertility journey, engage in mindfulness and present-moment awareness exercises. Pay attention to the present moment rather than ruminating on the past or fretting about the future. Accept the path as it takes you, having faith in the natural intelligence of your body and the sequence of events that make up life.

Adorn Yourself with Positive Encounters: Make sure you are in the company of uplifting situations, encouraging interactions, and good influences that will boost your optimism and general well-being. Spend time with supportive and encouraging loved ones, look for motivational tales of successful conception, and participate in enjoyable, fulfilling activities.

Let Go of Attachment to Results: Remain detached and allow life to unfold naturally while having faith in the universe's divine wisdom and timing. Let go of your connection to certain results and approach the path with trust, curiosity, and openness. Give up strict expectations and make room for miracles to happen in ways you never imagined.

Seek Assistance and Relationships: Join support groups, online forums, or see fertility coaches or counselors to find others who can relate to and understand your experience with infertility. On your journey to conception, talking to others about your feelings, struggles, and experiences may provide you support, encouragement, and a feeling of community.

Honor minor victories: Savor each advancement, regardless of size, on your path to fertility. Recognize and appreciate your bravery, tenacity, and hard work in overcoming the obstacles and uncertainties associated with conception. Acknowledge your inner power and fortitude and the fact that every day is a chance for development, education, and change.

Chapter 5: Overcoming Challenges and Obstacles

- **Addressing Common Fertility Issues and Concerns**
- **Strategies for Managing Hormonal Imbalances**
- **Dealing with Polycystic Ovary Syndrome (PCOS) and Endometriosis**
- **Seeking Support and Guidance When Facing Infertility**

Addressing Common Fertility Issues and Concerns

For single people and couples trying for a child, overcoming obstacles related to infertility may be a difficult and emotionally draining process. Making educated decisions, practicing proactive management, and obtaining the right assistance all depend on having a thorough understanding of typical reproductive challenges and concerns.

The following list of typical fertility problems and solutions is provided:

Menstrual Cycle Disorders: Menstrual cycle irregularities may be a sign of thyroid problems, polycystic ovarian syndrome (PCOS), or other problems relating to reproductive health. Monitoring menstrual cycles and seeing a doctor may help determine the underlying problems and direct the course of therapy.

Disorders of Ovulation: Infertility may be exacerbated by ovulatory abnormalities such as anovulation or irregular ovulation. Regular ovulation may be supported by lifestyle changes like as eating a balanced diet, controlling stress, and keeping a healthy weight. In some situations, doctors may also prescribe drugs to induce ovulation, such as letrozole or clomiphene citrate.

Low Sperm Quality or Count: Male fertility may be impacted by low sperm count or poor sperm quality. Smoking, binge drinking, and exposure to pollutants in the environment are examples of lifestyle choices that might impact sperm function and production. Male infertility issues may be resolved by leading a healthy lifestyle, abstaining from drugs, and seeing a fertility professional.

Blockages in the tubules: Tubal blockages may clog the fallopian tubes, preventing sperm from accessing the egg or the fertilized egg from implanting in the uterus. These blockages are often caused by pelvic inflammatory disease, endometriosis, or past pelvic procedures. Surgical procedures such as tubal reanastomosis or in vitro fertilization (IVF) may be advised, depending on the location and severity of the obstruction.

Endometriosis: When endometrial-like tissue proliferates outside the uterus, it may lead to pelvic discomfort, inflammation, and infertility. This disease is known as endometriosis. Assisted reproductive technologies (ART) including IVF, hormone therapy, laparoscopic surgery to remove endometrial implants, and pain management techniques are some examples of treatment methods.

Age-Related Fertility Decline: The quality and number of eggs produced by older mothers might be affected, which raises the possibility of infertility and pregnancy problems. beyond age 35, fertility steadily decreases, and beyond age 40, it decreases more dramatically. It may be helpful for women who are thinking about becoming pregnant later in life to speak with a fertility professional about fertility preservation measures like egg freezing.

Unknown Cause of Infertility: Unexplained infertility is the term used to describe situations in which a couple has infertility without a discernible underlying reason. Treatment options include intrauterine insemination (IUI), IVF, timed intercourse, and lifestyle adjustments. The emotional difficulties of unexplained infertility may also be managed by individuals and couples with the aid of counseling and support programs.

Infertility due to Male and Female Factors: A woman may become infertile due to a male, female, or mixed reason. Comprehensive fertility tests, which include hormone assessments, imaging investigations, ovarian reserve testing, and semen analysis, may assist pinpoint contributory causes and provide individualized therapy regimens designed to address particular reproductive problems.

Effects on the mind and emotions: Difficulties with fertility may have a negative impact on mental health, resulting in stress, worry, despair, and bereavement. During the reproductive process, seeking assistance from mental health specialists, support groups, or counseling services may provide emotional validation, coping mechanisms, and a feeling of community.

Aspects of Finance: Financial factors may play a role in treatment choices for fertility disorders since these therapies may be costly. Examining available resources, funding choices, and insurance coverage may help reduce financial stress and make access to reproductive therapy easier.

Strategies for Managing Hormonal Imbalances

In both men and women, hormonal abnormalities have the potential to impair reproductive health and exacerbate fertility issues. Optimizing reproductive results and promoting general well-being may be achieved by putting hormone imbalance management measures into practice. The following are some practical methods for treating hormone imbalances:

Optimal Nutrition and Diet: Eat a well-balanced diet full of fruits, vegetables, lean meats, whole grains, and healthy fats. Include foods like leafy greens, cruciferous vegetables, fatty salmon, nuts, seeds, and legumes that promote hormone balance in your diet. Reduce your consumption of bad fats, processed meals, and refined sweets since they may exacerbate hormone abnormalities.

Frequent Workout: Regular exercise may help to maintain hormonal balance, lower stress levels, and improve general health. Include a range of physical activities, such as Pilates, yoga, strength training, and cardiovascular workouts. On most days of the week, try to get in at least 30 minutes of moderate-intensity exercise.

Techniques for Stress Management: Engage in stress-reduction practices such progressive muscle relaxation, yoga, tai chi, deep breathing exercises, and mindfulness meditation. Prolonged stress may throw off the hormonal balance by lowering fertility, changing reproductive hormones, and raising cortisol levels.

Sufficient Rest and Sleep: Make getting enough sleep and rest a priority to help with hormone control and general health. Set up a regular sleep pattern and try to get between seven and nine hours of good sleep every night. Establish a calming nighttime routine, minimize screen time before bed, and furnish your bedroom with suitable furnishings that promote sound sleep.

Minimize Your Endocrine Disruptor Exposure: Minimize your exposure to chemicals that disrupt hormones, such as those contained in plastics, pesticides, cleaning supplies, and personal hygiene items. When feasible, use natural cleaning supplies, organic vegetables, and BPA-free plastics. When storing food, use glass or stainless steel containers; do not microwave plastics.

Sustain a Healthy Weight: Reach and stay at a healthy weight by eating a well-balanced diet and doing frequent exercise. Obesity—particularly fat around the abdomen—can aggravate insulin resistance, hormone abnormalities, and reproductive problems. For your age and height, try to keep your body mass index (BMI) within a healthy range.

Balanced Hormone Supplements: Vitamins, minerals, and herbal supplements that promote reproductive health and hormone balance should be taken into consideration. A healthcare professional or fertility expert may advise you on the right supplements depending on your requirements and current health. Vitamin D, omega-3 fatty acids, magnesium, zinc, and herbal supplements including chasteberry (Vitex) and maca root are common supplements for hormone balance.

Medical Care and Hormone Replacement Therapy: Medical care and hormone therapy may be required in situations of identified hormonal abnormalities, such as polycystic ovarian syndrome (PCOS), thyroid conditions, or male hypogonadism. Create a customized treatment plan in collaboration with an endocrinologist or healthcare professional to address underlying hormone imbalances and improve reproductive results.

Frequent observation and follow-up: Keep an eye on your hormone levels and reproductive health by scheduling routine checkups, blood tests, and fertility assessments. Keep track of your ovulation cycles, menstruation cycles, and any changes in your symptoms or worries about fertility. Hormonal abnormalities may be quickly identified and treated with the assistance of open conversation with healthcare experts.

Integrative medicine and holistic methods: To promote hormone balance and reproductive health, investigate integrative treatments and holistic techniques including acupuncture, chiropractic care, traditional Chinese medicine (TCM), and naturopathic medicine. These alternative therapies may enhance traditional medical care and improve general health.

Dealing with Polycystic Ovary Syndrome (PCOS) and Endometriosis

Polycystic Ovary Syndrome (PCOS) and endometriosis are two common gynecological conditions that can impact fertility and reproductive health in women. Managing PCOS and endometriosis requires a comprehensive approach that addresses symptoms, hormonal imbalances, and fertility concerns. Here are strategies for dealing with PCOS and endometriosis:

Understanding PCOS:

- PCOS is a hormonal disorder characterized by irregular menstrual cycles, ovarian cysts, and hormonal imbalances. Common symptoms include irregular periods, ovarian cysts, acne, hirsutism (excess hair growth), and weight gain.

- Diagnosis is typically based on symptoms, physical examination, blood tests to measure hormone levels, and ultrasound imaging of the ovaries.

Managing PCOS Symptoms:

- Lifestyle modifications, including regular exercise, a balanced diet, and weight management, can help improve insulin sensitivity and hormone balance in women with PCOS.

- Medications such as oral contraceptives, anti-androgen medications, and insulin-sensitizing agents may be prescribed to regulate menstrual cycles, reduce androgen levels, and manage symptoms.

- Fertility medications, such as clomiphene citrate or letrozole, may be used to induce ovulation in women with PCOS who are trying to conceive.

Addressing Endometriosis:

- Endometriosis is a condition in which tissue similar to the lining of the uterus grows outside the uterus, causing inflammation, pain, and scarring. Common symptoms include pelvic pain, painful periods, painful intercourse, and infertility.

- Diagnosis is often based on symptoms, pelvic examination, imaging studies, such as ultrasound or MRI, and laparoscopic surgery to visualize and biopsy endometrial tissue.

Managing Endometriosis Symptoms:

- Pain management strategies, including over-the-counter pain relievers, nonsteroidal anti-inflammatory drugs (NSAIDs), and prescription medications, can help alleviate pelvic pain and discomfort associated with endometriosis.

- Hormonal therapies, such as oral contraceptives, progestins, gonadotropin-releasing hormone (GnRH) agonists, or danazol, may be prescribed to suppress menstruation, reduce endometrial growth, and alleviate symptoms.

- Surgical interventions, such as laparoscopic excision or ablation of endometrial lesions, may be recommended to remove abnormal tissue and improve fertility outcomes.

Fertility Considerations:

- Both PCOS and endometriosis can impact fertility by affecting ovulation, egg quality, and implantation. Women with PCOS may benefit from ovulation induction medications, while those with endometriosis may require surgical interventions or assisted reproductive technologies (ART) such as in vitro fertilization (IVF).

- In vitro fertilization (IVF) may be recommended for couples struggling with infertility due to PCOS, endometriosis, or both conditions. IVF involves the retrieval of eggs from the ovaries, fertilization with sperm in a laboratory setting, and transfer of embryos into the uterus.

Holistic Approaches and Lifestyle Modifications:

- Integrative therapies, such as acupuncture, chiropractic care, herbal medicine, and dietary supplements, may complement conventional treatments and help manage symptoms of PCOS and endometriosis.

- Adopting a healthy lifestyle, including regular exercise, stress management techniques, and a balanced diet rich in fruits, vegetables, whole grains, and lean proteins, can support hormonal balance, reduce inflammation, and promote overall well-being.

Seeking Support and Advocacy:

- Connect with support groups, online communities, and advocacy organizations for PCOS and endometriosis to find support, resources, and information. Share experiences, insights, and challenges with others who understand and empathize with your journey.

- Dealing with PCOS and endometriosis requires a multidisciplinary approach that addresses symptoms, hormonal imbalances, fertility concerns, and emotional well-being. Working closely with healthcare providers, fertility specialists, and support networks can help individuals navigate the challenges of these conditions and optimize fertility

outcomes while promoting overall health
and quality of life.

Seeking Support and Guidance When Facing Infertility

It may be emotionally taxing and lonely to deal with infertility, but along the way, asking for help and advice can provide consolation, affirmation, and empowerment. Here are a few strategies for getting help while dealing with infertility:

Speak with Your Loved Ones: Talk to loved ones, relatives, or trustworthy friends about your emotions, ideas, and experiences. By sharing your infertility challenges with people closest to you, you may reduce feelings of loneliness and encourage compassion and understanding.

Participate in Support Groups: Take into consideration attending online or in-person infertility support groups. Making connections with others who are experiencing comparable things may give you a feeling of camaraderie, validation, and support. Online discussion boards and support groups provide a secure environment for exchanging personal experiences, asking queries, and getting assistance from others who are cognizant of your struggles.

Attend therapy or counseling: Seek assistance from mental health specialists who provide treatment or counseling for infertility. You may process difficult emotions, create coping mechanisms, and face the difficulties of infertility head-on with resilience and fortitude with the support of counseling. Therapy may provide a secure and accepting environment for discussing sorrow, loss, anxiety, and sadness associated with infertility.

Make Contact with Experts in Fertility: To learn more about treatment choices, fertility tests, and reproductive health treatments, speak with infertility clinics, reproductive endocrinologists, or fertility experts. Fertility experts may provide you with individualized advice, professional medical knowledge, and evidence-based therapies that are specific to your requirements and situation.

Examine Alternative Medical Interventions: Examine complementary and alternative treatments, like acupuncture, massage therapy, chiropractic adjustments, and naturopathic medicine, when it comes to conception. These complementary treatments have the potential to improve reproductive results, lower stress levels, and enhance general well-being.

Learn for Yourself: Spend some time learning about reproductive health, infertility, and the many treatment choices. Keep up with the most recent findings, developments in the field of reproductive science, and alternate methods of providing reproductive care. Having knowledge gives you the ability to speak up for what you need, make wise choices, and take an active role in your reproductive process.

Take Care of Yourself: As you work through the difficulties of infertility, give your mental and physical health first priority. Take part in enjoyable, stress-relieving, and fulfilling activities; they might include hobbies, physical activity, artistic endeavors, and time spent in nature. Establish limits in stressful circumstances and give your own well-being first priority.

Depend on Your Companion: During the reproductive process, rely on your spouse for understanding, emotional support, and camaraderie. Share your thoughts, concerns, and aspirations for the future in an honest and open manner. Together, provide love, empathy, and steadfast support to one another as you navigate the highs and lows of infertility.

Request Financial Support: To lessen the cost burden of fertility treatments and reproductive interventions, look into financial assistance programs, insurance coverage, and fertility finance possibilities. To make reproductive therapy more accessible and inexpensive, a lot of fertility clinics provide financing alternatives, reduced packages, and payment plans.

Remain upbeat and resilient: Navigate the unknowns and difficulties of infertility by holding onto hope, fortitude, and optimism. Have faith in your capacity to overcome challenges, endure hardships, and welcome the prospect of fresh starts. Hold on to your inner fortitude, faith, and conviction that miracles are possible.

Chapter 6: Partner Support and Collaboration

- **The Role of Partners in the Preconception Journey**
- **Encouraging Open Communication and Mutual Support**
- **Exploring Fertility Treatments and Assisted Reproductive Technologies**
- **Strengthening Your Relationship Through the Fertility Journey**

The Role of Partners in the Preconception Journey

Preconception requires active involvement and support from both partners in a relationship, rather than being the exclusive duty of one couple. In order to maximize reproductive health, foster a fertile environment, and be ready for parenting, partners are essential. Partners may help with the preconception journey in the following ways:

Honest Communication: Encourage couples to communicate honestly and openly about their hopes, worries, and aspirations for creating a family. It is possible for couples to connect their objectives and provide support to one another throughout the preconception journey by talking about family planning goals, fertility ambitions, and anticipated problems.

Endorsing Changes in Lifestyle: Encourage and assist one another in embracing a healthy lifestyle that supports reproductive health and fertility. To improve general health and fertility results, partners should work together on diet planning, exercise regimens, stress management strategies, and good sleep patterns.

Getting to medical appointments in tandem: Go to doctor's visits, fertility tests, and reproductive health checks together. During the preconception phase, partner participation in fertility consultations, diagnostic testing, and treatment conversations promotes understanding between the partners, joint decision-making, and emotional support.

Distributing Accountabilities: Assign duties to each other for measuring fertility, keeping an eye on ovulation, and implementing reproductive health measures. In order to maximize the timing of conception, partners might work together on techniques for fertility awareness, menstrual cycle monitoring, and the identification of viable windows.

Giving Emotional Assistance: Encourage one another, show empathy, and provide emotional support to one another amid the highs and lows of the preconception journey. Provide a secure environment for candid communication and vulnerability by validating one another's feelings, anxieties, and worries.

Overcoming Obstacles Together: As a team, overcome obstacles and setbacks, encouraging one another through infertility problems, losses, and uncertainty. During trying circumstances, partners may rely on one another for support, resiliency, and strength.

Honoring Significant Occasions and Triumphs: Honor significant junctures, triumphs, and happy times along the preconception journey. Recognize one another's perseverance, hard work, and contributions to the common goal of establishing a family.

Getting Knowledge About Fertility: Become knowledgeable about preconception care, fertility, and reproductive health. To maximize the results of fertility, partners may educate themselves about the variables affecting fertility, the time of ovulation, the significance of nutritional assistance, and lifestyle changes.

Addressing Intimacy and Sexual Health: Put your partner's sexual well-being and intimacy first while keeping lines of communication open and your bond strong. Couples might investigate methods for improving closeness, strengthening emotional ties, and creating a supportive atmosphere for conception.

Seeking Expert Assistance When Required: When dealing with fertility issues or seeking preconception care, see reproductive endocrinologists, counselors, or fertility experts for expert advice and assistance. In order to investigate treatment choices, resolve issues, and negotiate the complexity of the preconception journey, partners might work in tandem with healthcare practitioners.

In the preconception journey, partners are essential because they provide love, support, and companionship to one another as they start the road towards motherhood. Partners may build a solid foundation for fertility, conception, and the joys of motherhood ahead by cooperating as a team, being transparent with one another, and taking care of their relationship.

Encouraging Open Communication and Mutual Support

One of the most important foundations of a successful and healthy preconception journey is open communication between partners. When a couple decides to become parents, having open communication and providing constant support may help to improve fertility, enhance the quality of their relationship, and prepare them for the rewarding experience of starting a family. Here's how to promote candid dialogue and assistance between people:

Establish a Secure and Judgmental Environment: Provide a space where both partners are comfortable sharing their ideas, emotions, and worries without fear of repercussions. Promote nonjudgmental dialogue and attentive listening so that people may open up to one another without worrying about being rejected or criticized.

Start Frequent Check-Ins: Set up specific periods for frequent check-ins and discussions on the preconception process. Make sure that both parties feel heard, understood, and supported by using this time to talk about the objectives, progress, difficulties, and feelings related to conception.

Engage in Active Listening: Give each other your undivided attention and empathy throughout talks to demonstrate active listening. Try to comprehend your partner's point of view, acknowledge their emotions, and answer in a kind and considerate manner. Refrain from interjecting or making snap judgments so that genuine comprehension and connection may develop.

Clarify your expectations and needs: Be open and honest about your goals, needs, and wishes for the preconception process. To promote mutual understanding and goal alignment, be clear in your communication with your spouse about your wishes, limits, and concerns.

Recognize and Accept Emotions: Acknowledge the gamut of emotions that might surface throughout the preconception journey and validate each other's feelings, including excitement, worry, disappointment, and optimism. Acknowledge each other's experiences and viewpoints with empathy, assurance, and affirmation.

Equitably Assign Responsibilities: Assign equally to each spouse the duties and obligations associated with preconception care, fertility monitoring, and lifestyle adjustments. Work together to make decisions, create plans of action, and implement corrective actions while making sure that each person feels empowered and participated in the process.

Provide Unrestricted Assistance: Throughout the preconception journey, provide your spouse constant encouragement, support, and unity. In times of doubt, difficulty, or adversity, be a source of encouragement, strength, and optimism, proving your dedication to the common goal of beginning a family.

Honor accomplishments and landmarks: Honor any and all victories, landmarks, and advancements accomplished along the preconception journey. Celebrate and respect one another's efforts, resiliency, and contributions to the common goal of creating a family, encouraging an attitude of thankfulness and appreciation in your partnership.

Seek Expert Advice in Concert: When it comes to the preconception journey, work together to seek expert counsel and support when necessary. As a team, attend doctor visits, fertility consultations, and counseling sessions to show support and cooperation while addressing reproductive health issues and fertility obstacles.

Take Care of Your Partnership: Throughout the preconception process, give your relationship's health and stability top priority. As you get ready to become parents, make time for intimacy, connection, and quality time spent together. This will strengthen the emotional relationship and trust between couples.

<u>**Exploring Fertility Treatments and Assisted Reproductive Technologies**</u>

For people and couples who are having trouble becoming pregnant, assisted reproductive technologies (ART) and fertility treatments provide alternatives and hope for them to realize their desire of becoming parents. These therapies, which range from simple interventions to complex operations, are designed to maximize fertility, address obstacles to reproduction, and make conception easier. An outline of popular fertility therapies and ART choices is provided below:

Induction of Ovulation: Ovulation induction is the process of stimulating ovulation in women with irregular or nonexistent menstrual cycles by administering drugs such as letrozole or clomiphene citrate. By causing the ovaries to produce mature eggs and regulating hormone levels, these drugs improve the likelihood of pregnancy.

IUI, or intrauterine insemination: During ovulation, concentrated and cleansed sperm are inserted directly into the uterus during intrauterine insemination, often referred to as artificial insemination. By avoiding possible obstacles to conception, IUI is often used to treat male factor infertility, cervical problems, or infertility that cannot be explained.

IVF, or in vitro fertilization: The intricate fertility procedure known as "in vitro fertilization" involves removing eggs from the ovaries, fertilizing them with sperm in a lab, and then transferring the developed embryos into the uterus. For a number of infertility issues, such as endometriosis, reduced ovarian reserve, tubal factor infertility, and infertility without apparent cause, IVF may be advised.

Injecting sperm intracytoplasmically (ICSI): A specific procedure called intracytoplasmic sperm injection is performed in combination with in vitro fertilization (IVF) to address male factor infertility. In order to aid in fertilization, a single sperm is injected straight into the cytoplasm of an egg during ICSI. Men who have low sperm counts, poor motility, or aberrant sperm morphology may benefit from this therapy.

Freezing-based cryopreservation of embryos: The process of freezing and storing extra embryos created during an IVF cycle for later use is known as embryo cryopreservation. Future IVF rounds may benefit from the flexibility and alternatives provided by frozen embryos, which can be preserved forever and thawed for transfer.

Donor Sperm or Eggs: In situations involving severe male or female infertility, genetic abnormalities, or advanced maternal age, donor eggs or sperm may be used. Donor gametes are taken from anonymous, vetted donors and utilized with in vitro fertilization (IVF) to create pregnancy.

Using a surrogate: Using a gestational carrier to carry and deliver a pregnancy on behalf of intended parents is known as surrogacy. Using the genetic material of the intending parents or donor gametes, an embryo is produced in a gestational surrogate and transferred to the surrogate's uterus for implantation and pregnancy.

Genetic testing prior to implantation (PGT): Before embryos are implanted during IVF, preimplantation genetic testing is a diagnostic process used to check for genetic anomalies, chromosomal problems, or hereditary illnesses. PGT lessens the chance that kids may have genetic problems by assisting in the identification of embryos with the best chance of implantation.

Preserving Fertility: Through fertility preservation methods, such as sperm banking and egg freezing (oocyte cryopreservation), people may save their potential for reproduction for a later time. Patients receiving treatments like chemotherapy, radiation therapy, or surgery that may impact fertility may want to think about fertility preservation.

Alternative & Complementary Medicines: In order to maximize results, lessen stress, and enhance general wellbeing, complementary and alternative therapies such as acupuncture, herbal medicine, nutritional supplements, and mind-body techniques may be used with traditional reproductive treatments.

Strengthening Your Relationship Through the Fertility Journey

Although the process of becoming pregnant may be emotionally draining and difficult, it also offers couples the chance to grow closer, strengthen their bond, and develop resilience as a unit. Working together to overcome obstacles related to infertility calls for tolerance, compassion, and steadfast support for one another. The following are some methods to make your connection stronger while going through the reproductive journey:

Honest and transparent communication: Encourage frank and open dialogue with your spouse about your ideas, emotions, and worries about infertility difficulties. Establish a secure environment where people can communicate, actively listen, and understand one another. This will enable people to share their experiences and express their feelings without fear of retribution.

Cooperative Decision-Making: Include your spouse in the choices you make about family planning, therapies for infertility, and other reproductive health issues. Work together to develop treatment plans, consider your alternatives, and come to conclusions that are consistent with your common values, objectives, and ambitions.

Validation & Empathy: Recognize the gamut of emotions your spouse may experience during the fertility process and provide understanding and affirmation for their sentiments. Provide comfort and support by reassuring them that their experiences are genuine and by demonstrating your empathy and sympathy.

Collaboration and Support for One Another: As a team, approach the fertility journey, encouraging one another through the highs and lows, successes and setbacks, doubts and difficulties. Provide your spouse with support, inspiration, and unity by exhibiting your steadfast dedication to overcoming hardships together.

Handle Stress in Concert: Make self-care and stress reduction strategies a priority in order to support both partners' emotional resilience and well-being. In order to create a feeling of balance and tranquility throughout the reproductive process, partake in stress-relieving and relaxation-promoting activities like exercise, mindfulness meditation, nature walks, or creative endeavors.

Honor minor victories: No matter how tiny the victory, milestone, or happy occasion may appear, it is important to celebrate them along the way to fertility. Respect and acknowledge each other's perseverance, hard work, and contributions to the common goal of starting a family in order to foster an attitude of thankfulness and appreciation in your partnership.

Preserve intimacy and closeness: Amidst the difficulties of infertility, place a high priority on intimacy and connection in your relationship by fostering physical affection, emotional closeness, and romantic gestures. Allocate time for intimate moments, romantic evenings, and cooperative pursuits that enhance and reinforce your relationship.

Seek Assistance Collectively: Rely on one another for assistance and, if necessary, seek expert advice and therapy together. As a team, attend therapy sessions, support groups, and fertility clinics to show solidarity and togetherness while overcoming emotional issues and reproductive challenges.

Develop Your Resilience and Patience: Develop resilience, patience, and optimism as you work through the many unknowns and intricate aspects of the reproductive process. Accept adversities as chances for development, education, and connection building, and have faith in your capacity to conquer them as a team with grace and tenacity.

Honor your partnership: In the middle of the reproductive journey, take some time to celebrate and treasure your relationship, acknowledging the love, devotion, and companionship that help you get through the difficult times in life. Give thanks for each other's presence, encouragement, and steadfast commitment to enduring the storms together.

Chapter 7: Embracing Fertility Enlightenment

- **Cultivating a Positive and Empowered Mindset**
- **Embracing the Journey of Conception with Grace and Patience**
- **Trusting in the Wisdom of Your Body and Its Natural Rhythms**
- **Finding Joy and Fulfillment Beyond Conception**

Cultivating a Positive and Empowered Mindset

The process of becoming pregnant may be emotionally taxing and full of unknowns, but people can handle the ups and downs with grace, resilience, and optimism by developing an empowered and optimistic mentality. Through proactive and positive approaches to the reproductive process, people may develop emotional stability, inner strength, and a feeling of empowerment. Throughout the process of becoming pregnant, consider the following techniques for developing an optimistic and strong mindset:

Exercise Self-Compassion: Throughout the process of becoming pregnant, remember to treat yourself with kindness and gentleness and understand that being infertile does not diminish your value as a person. When you feel frustrated, disappointed, or self-conscious, particularly, remember to treat yourself with understanding, tolerance, and acceptance. This is an example of practicing self-compassion.

Concentrate on What You Can Manage: Turn your attention to the areas of the reproductive process that you can influence, such lifestyle decisions, self-care routines, and mental health. Invest your efforts in preventative steps that enhance general health and fertility, giving you the confidence to make wise decisions.

Have Reasonable Expectations: Have reasonable expectations for the reproductive process, understanding that things may not go as planned and that things could happen slowly. Accept the trip as a process of resilience, development, and learning, and make room for acceptance, flexibility, and adaptability along the way.

Practice Being Present and Mindful: Develop present-moment awareness and mindfulness to enable yourself to completely experience and welcome the adventure as it happens. Resolve your concerns about the past and future by centering yourself in the present now via mindful breathing, meditation, or grounding techniques.

Make Your Dreams and Goals Visible: Use visualization exercises to picture your hopes, desires, and objectives for starting a family. Building a vision board, keeping a diary of your ideas and emotions, or visualizing successful results are all ways to cultivate hope, optimism, and potential in your heart and mind.

Seek Guidance and Assistance: As you embark on your fertility journey, surround yourself with people who will inspire, motivate, and support you. Create a feeling of solidarity and connection with others who understand your path by getting in touch with support groups, online communities, or inspiring materials that align with your values, beliefs, and objectives.

Honor minor victories: Acknowledge and respect any progress accomplished, no matter how modest, by celebrating minor triumphs, significant anniversaries, and happy moments along the way to fertility. Recognize your fortitude, bravery, and tenacity in the face of difficulties while developing an attitude of thankfulness and appreciation for all the gifts in your life.

Practice Positive Self-Talk and Affirmations: As you traverse the reproductive path, remind yourself of your power, resilience, and worthiness by including affirmations and positive self-talk into your daily routine. An attitude of confidence and self-belief may be fostered by substituting positive words that empower and elevate you for negative ideas and self-doubt.

Take Part in Intentional Activities: Beyond the process of becoming pregnant, take part in things that make you happy, fulfilled, and feel like you have a purpose. Remind yourself of the depth and wealth that exist in your life outside of reproductive issues by pursuing activities, passions, and hobbies that feed your soul and spark your creativity.

Accept the Force of Hope: Accept the ability of hope to keep you going through the highs and lows of your reproductive journey. Have a steadfast faith in the potential for miracles, fresh starts, and unforeseen benefits. Have faith in the human spirit's innate fortitude and the process of becoming a parent.

<u>**Embracing the Journey of Conception with Grace and Patience**</u>

The process of becoming pregnant is a very intimate and life-changing event that has its own pace, difficulties, and rewards. Individuals and couples may handle the ups and downs of fertility with resilience, optimism, and serenity if they approach this path with kindness and patience. Here are some strategies for accepting the conception process with patience and grace:

Foster Acceptance: Accept the way that the reproductive journey is playing out right now, without opposition or condemnation. Acknowledge that obstacles and disappointments are a part of the process, and as you go along the road to motherhood, cultivate self-compassion and understanding.

Have faith in the divine timing: Have faith in the natural rhythms of conception and the wisdom of divine timing, understanding that every person's path follows a distinct course. Give up control over the results and have faith that the universe has a purpose for your path, even if that purpose is not what you had in mind.

Develop Your Surrender and Patience: When faced with uncertainty and waiting, practice patience and surrender. Have faith that everything is happening in due time and that patience is a virtue that makes room for development, resiliency, and the eventual manifestation of benefits.

Concentrate on the Here and Now: Savor the experiences, pleasures, and joys that come with being fertile by being centered in the here and now. Notwithstanding any obstacles or doubts that may come up, practice mindfulness and an appreciation of the wonder and beauty that are present in every moment.

Boost Your Emotional Health: Make self-care routines that nourish your heart, mind, and soul a priority, along with your emotional well-being. Take part in joyful, peaceful, and fulfilling activities; these might include spending time in nature, doing yoga or meditation, or spending time with supportive and inspiring family members.

Honor minor victories: Savor the little triumphs, significant anniversaries, and happy moments that arise throughout the conception process. Recognize and respect your fortitude, bravery, and resolve in meeting obstacles head-on and accepting the journey with appreciation and grace.

Seek Assistance and Relationships: Seek out relationships and support from family, friends, or support groups that have experienced similar things as you. Openly express your ideas, emotions, and experiences while keeping in mind that you are not alone and that connection and vulnerability breed strength.

Sustain your optimism and hope: Develop optimism and hope as guiding principles to help you get through the highs and lows of the reproductive journey. Maintain an open mind to the possibility of miracles, blessings, and fresh starts. Have faith in the ability of hope to light the way ahead.

Expectations and Attachments of Release: Let go of expectations or attachments to certain results about the course of the conception process. Let go of your fixed expectations and narrow mindset to make room in your life for miracles, unexpected benefits, and spiritual direction.

Exercise appreciation and gratitude: Develop an attitude of thankfulness and appreciation for all the benefits, insights, and development that come with the journey of conception. Acknowledge the journey's beauty and holiness and welcome each encounter as a chance for growth, learning, and spiritual awareness.

It is a transformational and holy process that asks people and couples to submit to the wisdom of the cosmos, believe in divine timing, and welcome the journey with open hearts and minds—embracing the journey of conception with grace and patience. People may travel the fertility journey with grace, patience, and a profound feeling of calm by developing resilience, acceptance, and trust. They can also know that they are supported and led every step of the way.

Trusting in the Wisdom of Your Body and Its Natural Rhythms

A crucial component of the fertility journey is having faith in the knowledge of your body and its inherent cycles. You may traverse the process of conception with more knowledge, resilience, and trust by tuning into your body's intrinsic wisdom. Your body is carefully constructed to conceive, nourish, and support life. Here are some strategies for having faith in your body's inherent cycles and wisdom:

Recognize the Menstrual Cycle: Learn about the many stages of your menstrual cycle, such as the luteal phase, ovulation, follicular phase, and menstruation. Utilize a reproductive awareness technique, fertility app, or calendar to track your cycle and spot trends and windows of opportunity for conception.

Pay Attention to Your Body's Cues: Pay attention to the subtle signs and indications your body sends out throughout the menstrual cycle, such as variations in cervical position, basal body temperature, and cervical mucus. Honoring your body's knowledge and insights, pay attention to bodily sensations, energy levels, and emotional swings.

Respecting Your Gut Feeling: Develop a closer relationship with your inner knowledge and intuition by having faith in the instinctive wisdom that emerges from inside. When deciding on fertility treatments, lifestyle options, and mental health, pay attention to your gut feelings, inner wisdom, and intuition cues.

Enhance Natural Fertility Health: Make holistic approaches—eating nutritious foods, drinking enough water, exercising often, controlling stress, and placing a high value on restful sleep—your top priorities when it comes to naturally enhancing your fertility. Accept lifestyle changes that promote reproductive health, hormone balance, and general wellbeing.

Have Faith in the Ability of Relaxation and Rest: Recognize how crucial rest and relaxation are to maintaining your body's normal cycles and the health of your fertility. Make time in your daily schedule for relaxation techniques that help your body decompress, rejuvenate, and regain equilibrium. These techniques include deep breathing, yoga, meditation, and spending time in nature.

Accept Nature's Healing Power: Spend time outside in the sunshine, crisp air, and natural surroundings to connect with the restorative power of nature. Take part in soul-nourishing activities that strengthen your connection with the planet, including hiking, gardening, or just taking in the beauty of nature.

Boost Your Emotional Health: Develop resilience and emotional well-being by fostering wholesome connections, partaking in happy and fulfilling pursuits, and asking for help when you need it. Develop self-care routines that respect your emotional needs and help you feel at ease, accepted, and in love with yourself.

Give Up Control and Give In: Give up trying to control every part of the process and let life unfold naturally. Have faith that the universe's wisdom will guide the blossoming of benefits and the divine timing of conception. Open yourself up to the trip, give yourself up to it, and have faith in your body's innate wisdom.

Appreciate the Power and Resilience of Your Body: Honor your body's tenacity, fortitude, and vigor as it supports you on your reproductive journey. Respect the amazing powers of your reproductive system and the wonder of the possibility of conception and the birth of new life.

Develop An Gratitude and Appreciation Culture: Acknowledge and respect your body and its natural cycles, and acknowledge the holiness and beauty of the reproductive process. Give thanks for your body's complex mechanisms, your gift of fertility, and the chance to co-create life with the cosmos.

One potent technique that asks you to submit to the intrinsic knowledge and direction that dwells within you is trusting in the wisdom of your body and its natural cycles. You may develop a closer relationship with yourself, your fertility, and the wonder of life that grows inside of you by respecting your body, paying attention to its signals, and welcoming the journey with trust and openness.

Finding Joy and Fulfillment Beyond Conception

It's crucial to understand that happiness and contentment are not limited to motherhood, even while the process of becoming pregnant may be profoundly meaningful and transformational. Regardless of the success or failure of infertility treatments, people and couples may build contentment, meaning, and pleasure in many facets of their life by adopting a holistic approach to well-being. Beyond conception, you may experience happiness and pleasure in the following ways:

Create Deeply Meaningful Relationships: Develop deep relationships with family, friends, and neighbors that encourage and assist you on your path. Make spending time with loved ones a priority in order to create a feeling of connection, belonging, and emotional support.

Follow your purpose and passion: Investigate your hobbies, interests, and skills, and engage in pursuits that give your life meaning and happiness. Take part in artistic efforts, volunteer work, professional endeavors, or pastimes that make you happy and that reflect your ideals.

Invest in Your Own Development: Embrace chances for learning, exploration, and self-improvement. Make a commitment to continuous personal progress and self-discovery. Participate in therapy sessions, seminars, or workshops that promote your psychological, spiritual, and emotional health and provide you the tools you need to grow and change as a person.

Practice Being Present and Mindful: Savor the richness and beauty of every moment as it comes to pass by practicing mindfulness and present in your day-to-day activities. To cultivate inner calm and clarity, try writing, deep breathing, or mindfulness meditation as ways to bring oneself into the present moment.

Investigate Outdoor Activities and Nature: Spend time outside in the sunshine, crisp air, and natural surroundings to connect with the restorative power of nature. Take part in outdoor pursuits like hiking, gardening, or stargazing, and let the natural world uplift and nurture your spirit.

Exercise appreciation and gratitude: Make it a daily habit to express your thanks and appreciation for all the richness, happiness, and blessings in your life. Maintain a thankfulness diary, show appreciation for the little things in life, and recognize the magic and beauty that you are surrounded by every day.

Put your health and wellbeing first: Make your mental, emotional, and physical health your top priority by forming wholesome lifestyle choices that promote general energy and wellness. To maximize your well-being, fuel your body with wholesome meals, drink enough water, exercise often, and give yourself enough restful sleep.

Accept Expression and Creativity: Accept your inner artist and develop your ability to express yourself via writing, music, painting, or other creative endeavors. Give yourself permission to explore and communicate your ideas, emotions, and experiences in a manner that is authentic to your voice and vision.

Seek Harmony and Balance: Aim for harmony and balance in all facets of your life, respecting the connection between the body, mind, and spirit. Establish limits, control your stress, and prioritize self-care to promote balance and wellbeing in your everyday routines.

Honor accomplishments and landmarks: Honor the strides you've made and the resiliency you've shown by celebrating your life's turning points, victories, and growth moments. Recognize your abilities, contributions to the world, and skills while appreciating and enjoying the ride.

Embracing the whole of life's experiences, welcoming the journey with an open heart, and discovering meaning and purpose in every moment are all necessary steps toward achieving pleasure and contentment beyond comprehension. Through fostering relationships, following interests, and promoting overall well being, individuals and couples may find deep happiness and contentment that surpasses the desire for motherhood.

Part Two

:

Fertility Kitchen

:

The Dietary Approach

Chapter 1: Understanding Fertility Nutrition

- **Exploring the Link Between Nutrition and Fertility**
- **Essential Nutrients for Fertility: Vitamins, Minerals, and Antioxidants**
- **Hormonal Balance and Fertility: The Role of Food**
- **Tips for Building a Fertility-Friendly Diet**

Exploring the Link Between Nutrition and Fertility

Nutrition plays a crucial role in reproductive health and fertility, influencing hormonal balance, egg and sperm quality, and overall reproductive function. Making informed dietary choices and adopting a nutrient-rich diet can optimize fertility outcomes and support the body's natural ability to conceive. Here's an exploration of the link between nutrition and fertility:

Balancing Macronutrients: A balanced intake of macronutrients, including carbohydrates, proteins, and fats, is essential for hormonal regulation and reproductive function. Opt for complex carbohydrates such as whole grains, lean proteins like poultry, fish, and plant-based sources, and healthy fats from avocados, nuts, seeds, and olive oil.

Prioritizing Micronutrients: Micronutrients such as vitamins, minerals, and antioxidants play critical roles in fertility and reproductive health. Key micronutrients for fertility include folate, zinc, selenium, vitamin D, vitamin E, vitamin C, and omega-3 fatty acids. Incorporate a variety of nutrient-rich foods such as leafy greens, colorful fruits and vegetables, nuts, seeds, legumes, and seafood to ensure adequate intake.

Supporting Hormonal Balance: Certain nutrients, such as vitamin B6, vitamin E, magnesium, and zinc, help support hormonal balance and regulate menstrual cycles. Consuming foods rich in these nutrients, such as leafy greens, whole grains, nuts, seeds, and legumes, can help promote regular ovulation and optimize fertility.

Improving Egg and Sperm Quality: Antioxidants play a key role in protecting eggs and sperm from oxidative damage and improving their quality. Foods rich in antioxidants, such as berries, citrus fruits, dark leafy greens, nuts, seeds, and colorful vegetables, can help enhance fertility by supporting reproductive health and DNA integrity.

Maintaining a Healthy Weight: Maintaining a healthy weight is important for fertility, as both underweight and overweight conditions can negatively impact reproductive function. Aim for a balanced diet and regular physical activity to achieve and maintain a healthy weight, which can help regulate menstrual cycles, optimize hormone levels, and improve fertility outcomes.

Minimizing Processed Foods and Sugars: Processed foods, sugary snacks, and beverages high in refined sugars can disrupt hormonal balance, increase inflammation, and negatively impact fertility. Limit intake of processed foods and sugary treats, opting instead for whole, nutrient-dense foods that support reproductive health and overall well-being.

Hydration and Fertility: Staying hydrated is essential for optimal fertility and reproductive function. Adequate hydration supports cervical mucus production, which is important for sperm motility and transport. Aim to drink plenty of water throughout the day and incorporate hydrating foods such as fruits, vegetables, and herbal teas into your diet.

Managing Stress with Nutrition: Chronic stress can adversely affect fertility by disrupting hormonal balance and ovulation. Incorporating stress-reducing foods such as complex carbohydrates, lean proteins, and foods rich in magnesium and B vitamins can help support the body's stress response and promote emotional well-being.

Considering Dietary Supplements: In addition to a balanced diet, certain individuals may benefit from dietary supplements to address specific nutrient deficiencies or support fertility. Consult with a healthcare provider or fertility specialist to determine if supplementation with vitamins, minerals, or herbal supplements may be appropriate for your individual needs.

Individualized Approach: It's important to recognize that nutritional needs vary among individuals and may be influenced by factors such as age, genetics, underlying health conditions, and lifestyle factors. Consider working with a registered dietitian or nutritionist specializing in fertility to develop a personalized nutrition plan tailored to your unique needs and goals.

By exploring the link between nutrition and fertility and making informed dietary choices, individuals and couples can optimize reproductive health, enhance fertility outcomes, and support the body's natural ability to conceive. Embracing a nutrient-rich diet, maintaining a healthy lifestyle, and prioritizing emotional well-being can create a foundation for optimal fertility and pave the way for a healthy and fulfilling conception journey.

Essential Nutrients for Fertility: Vitamins, Minerals, and Antioxidants

Nutrition plays a crucial role in fertility, influencing reproductive health, hormone balance, and overall fertility outcomes. A well-balanced diet rich in essential nutrients can optimize fertility in both men and women, while poor dietary choices may impair reproductive function and fertility. Let's explore the key nutrients and their roles in promoting fertility:

Folic Acid (Folate): Folic acid is a B vitamin essential for DNA synthesis and cell division, making it critical for healthy egg and sperm development. Adequate folic acid intake before conception reduces the risk of neural tube defects in babies. Foods rich in folate include leafy greens, beans, lentils, fortified cereals, and citrus fruits.

Iron: Iron is essential for healthy blood production and oxygen transport throughout the body, including the reproductive organs. Iron deficiency anemia can impair ovulation and menstrual cycles in women and reduce sperm quality in men. Iron-rich foods include lean meats, poultry, fish, beans, lentils, spinach, and fortified cereals.

Omega-3 Fatty Acids: Omega-3 fatty acids, particularly EPA and DHA, support reproductive health by reducing inflammation, improving blood flow to the reproductive organs, and promoting hormone balance. Sources of omega-3 fatty acids include fatty fish (salmon, mackerel, sardines), flaxseeds, chia seeds, walnuts, and algae-based supplements.

Antioxidants: Antioxidants such as vitamins C and E, selenium, and zinc help protect reproductive cells from oxidative damage caused by free radicals. Antioxidants support sperm quality, egg health, and embryo development. Foods rich in antioxidants include berries, citrus fruits, nuts, seeds, leafy greens, and whole grains.

Vitamin D: Vitamin D plays a crucial role in reproductive health, hormone regulation, and immune function. Low vitamin D levels have been associated with infertility, irregular menstrual cycles, and poor sperm quality. Natural sources of vitamin D include sunlight exposure, fatty fish, fortified dairy products, and egg yolks.

B Vitamins: B vitamins, including B6, B12, and riboflavin (B2), are important for hormone balance, energy production, and DNA synthesis. Deficiencies in B vitamins can disrupt ovulation and impair sperm quality. Sources of B vitamins include whole grains, lean meats, poultry, fish, eggs, dairy products, and leafy greens.

Zinc: Zinc is essential for sperm production, testosterone synthesis, and egg maturation. Zinc deficiency can impair fertility and increase the risk of pregnancy complications. Good sources of zinc include lean meats, poultry, seafood, nuts, seeds, beans, and whole grains.

Magnesium: Magnesium plays a role in hundreds of biochemical reactions in the body, including DNA synthesis, muscle function, and hormone regulation. Adequate magnesium levels are important for reproductive health and fertility. Food sources of magnesium include leafy greens, nuts, seeds, whole grains, and legumes.

Protein: Protein is essential for building and repairing tissues, including reproductive tissues. Adequate protein intake supports hormone production, egg development, and sperm quality. Good sources of protein include lean meats, poultry, fish, eggs, dairy products, beans, lentils, and tofu.

Iodine: Iodine is crucial for thyroid function, metabolism, and hormone regulation, including reproductive hormones. Iodine deficiency can disrupt menstrual cycles and impair fertility. Dietary sources of iodine include iodized salt, seafood, seaweed, dairy products, and fortified grains.

Hormonal Balance and Fertility: The Role of Food

Achieving and maintaining hormonal balance is crucial for optimal fertility in both men and women. Hormones play a pivotal role in regulating reproductive processes, including ovulation, sperm production, and implantation. Diet and nutrition can significantly influence hormonal balance, either supporting or disrupting reproductive health. Here's an exploration of the role of food in hormonal balance and fertility:

Impact of Diet on Hormonal Regulation: The foods we consume provide the building blocks for hormone synthesis and metabolism. Certain nutrients, such as vitamins, minerals, and phytonutrients, play key roles in hormonal regulation and fertility. A diet rich in nutrient-dense foods can help support hormonal balance and optimize reproductive function.

Balancing Blood Sugar Levels: Consumption of refined carbohydrates and sugary foods can lead to fluctuations in blood sugar levels, which may disrupt hormonal balance and impair fertility. Choosing complex carbohydrates, high-fiber foods, and sources of healthy fats and proteins can help stabilize blood sugar levels and support hormonal health.

Importance of Essential Fatty Acids: Essential fatty acids, such as omega-3 and omega-6 fatty acids, are critical for hormone production and cellular function. Omega-3 fatty acids, found in fatty fish, flaxseeds, chia seeds, and walnuts, have anti-inflammatory properties and support reproductive health. Balancing omega-3 and omega-6 fatty acids is essential for maintaining hormonal equilibrium.

Role of Protein and Amino Acids: Protein-rich foods provide essential amino acids necessary for hormone synthesis and tissue repair. Consuming adequate amounts of high-quality protein sources, such as lean meats, poultry, fish, eggs, legumes, and dairy products, supports hormonal balance and fertility.

Antioxidants and Hormonal Health: Antioxidants play a crucial role in protecting reproductive cells from oxidative damage and supporting hormonal balance. Foods rich in antioxidants, including fruits, vegetables, nuts, seeds, and whole grains, help neutralize free radicals and reduce inflammation, supporting overall reproductive health.

Impact of Phytonutrients: Phytonutrients, found in colorful fruits, vegetables, and herbs, offer numerous health benefits, including hormonal balance. Phytonutrients such as flavonoids, polyphenols, and carotenoids have antioxidant and anti-inflammatory properties that support reproductive function and may help regulate hormone levels.

Role of Fiber and Gut Health: Fiber-rich foods support gut health and promote the elimination of excess hormones from the body. A healthy digestive system ensures proper absorption and metabolism of nutrients essential for hormonal balance. Incorporating fiber-rich foods such as fruits, vegetables, whole grains, and legumes into your diet can support hormonal health and fertility.

Limiting Exposure to Hormone Disruptors: Certain environmental toxins and endocrine-disrupting chemicals found in pesticides, plastics, and personal care products can interfere with hormonal balance and fertility. Choosing organic foods, minimizing exposure to toxins, and opting for natural, non-toxic household and personal care products can help reduce the risk of hormone disruption.

Maintaining a Healthy Weight: Maintaining a healthy body weight is important for hormonal balance and fertility. Both underweight and overweight conditions can disrupt hormone levels and impair reproductive function. Adopting a balanced diet, engaging in regular physical activity, and managing stress can support weight management and hormonal health.

Individualized Approach to Nutrition: It's important to recognize that nutritional needs vary among individuals, and there is no one-size-fits-all approach to optimizing hormonal balance and fertility. Consulting with a healthcare provider or registered dietitian can help assess individual nutritional needs, identify potential deficiencies or imbalances, and develop a personalized nutrition plan to support reproductive health.

<u>**Tips for Building a Fertility-Friendly Diet**</u>

Building a fertility-friendly diet involves focusing on nutrient-dense foods that support hormonal balance, reproductive health, and overall well-being. Here are some tips to help you create a diet that enhances fertility:

Balance Your Macronutrients: Ensure your meals include a balance of carbohydrates, proteins, and healthy fats. Whole grains, lean proteins, and sources of healthy fats like avocados, nuts, and seeds can help stabilize blood sugar levels and support hormone production.

Emphasize Plant-Based Foods: Load up on fruits, vegetables, legumes, and whole grains. These foods are rich in vitamins, minerals, antioxidants, and fiber, which can help regulate hormone levels and promote reproductive health.

Choose Healthy Proteins: Incorporate lean sources of protein such as poultry, fish, beans, lentils, and tofu into your meals. Protein is essential for cell growth and repair, hormone production, and overall reproductive health.

Include Omega-3 Fatty Acids: Omega-3 fatty acids found in fatty fish like salmon, walnuts, flaxseeds, and chia seeds are beneficial for fertility. They help reduce inflammation, support egg and sperm quality, and regulate hormone production.

Opt for Complex Carbohydrates: Choose complex carbohydrates such as whole grains, sweet potatoes, quinoa, and brown rice over refined carbohydrates. Complex carbs provide sustained energy, regulate blood sugar levels, and support hormone balance.

Prioritize Iron-Rich Foods: Iron is crucial for reproductive health and fertility. Include iron-rich foods such as lean red meat, poultry, fish, beans, lentils, spinach, and fortified cereals in your diet to prevent anemia and support fertility.

Get Plenty of Antioxidants: Antioxidant-rich foods help protect reproductive cells from damage caused by free radicals. Include colorful fruits and vegetables such as berries, citrus fruits, leafy greens, bell peppers, and carrots in your diet to boost antioxidant intake.

Limit Processed Foods and Added Sugars: Processed foods and foods high in added sugars can disrupt hormone balance and contribute to inflammation. Opt for whole, minimally processed foods whenever possible, and limit your intake of sugary snacks and beverages.

Stay Hydrated: Drink plenty of water throughout the day to stay hydrated and support overall health. Hydration is essential for optimal hormonal function, nutrient absorption, and detoxification.

Moderate Caffeine and Alcohol Intake: Limit your consumption of caffeine and alcohol, as excessive intake may interfere with hormone levels and fertility. Opt for herbal teas, water, and occasional indulgences in moderation.

Maintain a Healthy Weight: Aim to maintain a healthy weight through balanced nutrition and regular physical activity. Both underweight and overweight can affect fertility and hormonal balance, so focus on achieving a healthy BMI (Body Mass Index).

Practice Mindful Eating: Pay attention to hunger and fullness cues, and practice mindful eating to foster a healthy relationship with food. Enjoy your meals slowly, savoring each bite, and listen to your body's signals of hunger and satisfaction.

By incorporating these tips into your daily diet, you can nourish your body, support fertility, and optimize your chances of conception. Remember, every small change can make a big difference on your fertility journey.

Chapter 2: Breakfasts for Fertility

- **Berry Blast Smoothie Bowl**
- **Avocado and Egg Breakfast Tacos**
- **Quinoa Porridge with Almond Milk and Berries**
- **Green Goddess Breakfast Salad**

<u>Berry Blast Smoothie Bowl</u>

Ingredients

- 1 cup mixed berries (such as strawberries, blueberries, raspberries)

- 1 ripe banana, sliced

- 1/2 cup plain Greek yogurt

- 1/4 cup almond milk (or your choice of milk)

- 1 tablespoon honey or maple syrup (optional, for sweetness)

- 1/4 cup granola

- 1 tablespoon chia seeds

- Fresh berries, sliced bananas, and mint leaves for garnish (optional)

Instructions

- In a blender, combine the mixed berries, sliced banana, Greek yogurt, almond milk, and honey or maple syrup (if using). Blend until smooth and creamy.

- Pour the smoothie mixture into a bowl.

- Sprinkle the granola and chia seeds evenly over the smoothie.

- Garnish with fresh berries, sliced bananas, and mint leaves if desired.

- Serve immediately and enjoy your refreshing and nutrient-packed Berry Blast Smoothie Bowl!

Note: Feel free to customize your smoothie bowl with additional toppings such as shredded coconut, nuts, seeds, or a drizzle of nut butter for added flavor and texture.

<u>**Avocado and Egg Breakfast Tacos**</u>

Gather Your Ingredients: Collect all the ingredients listed in the recipe - mixed berries (strawberries, blueberries, raspberries), a ripe banana, plain Greek yogurt, almond milk (or your preferred milk alternative), honey or maple syrup (optional), granola, chia seeds, and any additional toppings you prefer.

Blend the Smoothie: In a blender, combine the mixed berries, sliced banana, Greek yogurt, almond milk, and honey or maple syrup (if using). Blend the ingredients until you achieve a smooth and creamy consistency. Adjust the sweetness according to your preference by adding more honey or maple syrup if desired.

Prepare the Toppings: Measure out the granola and chia seeds for topping the smoothie bowl. You can also prepare additional toppings such as fresh berries, sliced bananas, mint leaves, shredded coconut, nuts, or seeds.

Assemble the Smoothie Bowl: Pour the blended smoothie mixture into a bowl, ensuring it's evenly distributed.

Add the Toppings: Sprinkle the granola and chia seeds evenly over the smoothie mixture in the bowl. Arrange the fresh berries, sliced bananas, and mint leaves on top for garnish and additional flavor.

Serve and Enjoy: Your Berry Blast Smoothie Bowl is now ready to be enjoyed! Serve it immediately to savor its refreshing taste and nutrient-packed goodness.

Feel free to get creative with your toppings and adjust the ingredients based on your preferences and dietary needs. Whether enjoyed as a nutritious breakfast, a satisfying snack, or a refreshing dessert, this smoothie bowl is sure to delight your taste buds and nourish your body with its vibrant flavors and wholesome ingredients.

Quinoa Porridge with Almond Milk and Berries

To prepare Quinoa Porridge with Almond Milk and Berries, follow these straightforward steps:

Ingredients

- 1/2 cup quinoa, rinsed

- 1 cup almond milk (or your preferred milk)

- 1/2 teaspoon ground cinnamon

- 1 tablespoon maple syrup or honey (optional, for sweetness)

- 1/4 cup mixed berries (such as strawberries, blueberries, raspberries)

- Sliced almonds or chopped nuts for topping (optional)

- Additional sweetener to taste (optional)

Instructions

Rinse the Quinoa: Before cooking, rinse the quinoa under cold water using a fine-mesh sieve to remove any bitterness.

Combine Quinoa and Almond Milk: In a small saucepan, combine the rinsed quinoa and almond milk. Add the ground cinnamon for flavor. Stir well to combine.

Cook the Quinoa: Place the saucepan over medium heat and bring the quinoa mixture to a gentle boil. Once boiling, reduce the heat to low and simmer uncovered for about 15-20 minutes, or until the quinoa is tender and the mixture has thickened to your desired consistency. Stir occasionally to prevent sticking.

Sweeten the Porridge: If desired, sweeten the quinoa porridge with maple syrup or honey. Adjust the sweetness according to your taste preferences. Stir well to incorporate the sweetener into the porridge.

Prepare the Berries: While the quinoa is cooking, wash and slice the berries for topping.

Serve the Quinoa Porridge: Once the quinoa is cooked to your liking and the porridge has reached your desired consistency, remove the saucepan from the heat. Allow the porridge to cool slightly before serving.

Assemble and Garnish: Spoon the quinoa porridge into serving bowls. Top each bowl with a generous serving of mixed berries and sliced almonds or chopped nuts for added texture and flavor.

Enjoy: Your Quinoa Porridge with Almond Milk and Berries is now ready to be enjoyed! Serve it warm and savor the comforting flavors of this nutritious breakfast dish.

Feel free to customize your quinoa porridge with additional toppings such as shredded coconut, chia seeds, or a drizzle of nut butter for added richness and variety. This wholesome breakfast option is packed with protein, fiber, and antioxidants, making it a nourishing way to start your day.

<u>**Green Goddess Breakfast Salad**</u>

To prepare a Green Goddess Breakfast Salad, you can follow these simple steps:

Ingredients

- 4 cups mixed greens (such as spinach, kale, arugula)

- 1 avocado, sliced

- 4 eggs

- 1 cup cherry tomatoes, halved

- 1/4 cup cucumber, sliced

- 1/4 cup red onion, thinly sliced

- 1/4 cup bell pepper, thinly sliced

- 1/4 cup feta cheese, crumbled (optional)

- 2 tablespoons fresh lemon juice

- 2 tablespoons extra-virgin olive oil

- Salt and pepper to taste

- **Optional toppings:** toasted seeds, nuts, or cooked quinoa

Instructions

Prepare the Eggs: You can prepare the eggs to your preference. For a breakfast salad, poached or soft-boiled eggs work well. Bring a pot of water to a gentle boil and carefully add the eggs. Cook for about 4-5 minutes for soft-boiled eggs or longer for firmer yolks. Once cooked, remove the eggs from the pot and place them in cold water to stop the cooking process. Peel the eggs and set them aside.

Prepare the Salad Base: Wash and dry the mixed greens thoroughly. Place them in a large salad bowl.

Add the Vegetables: Slice the avocado, cherry tomatoes, cucumber, red onion, and bell pepper. Add them to the salad bowl with the mixed greens.

Prepare the Dressing: In a small bowl, whisk together the fresh lemon juice, extra-virgin olive oil, salt, and pepper to create the dressing.

Assemble the Salad: Drizzle the dressing over the salad ingredients in the bowl. Gently toss everything together until the salad is evenly coated with the dressing.

Plate the Salad: Divide the dressed salad mixture into individual serving bowls or plates.

Add the Eggs and Optional Toppings: Place a poached or soft-boiled egg on top of each salad serving. Sprinkle crumbled feta cheese (if using) over the salads. You can also add additional toppings such as toasted seeds, nuts, or cooked quinoa for extra protein and texture.

Serve and Enjoy: Your Green Goddess Breakfast Salad is now ready to be served! Enjoy this vibrant and nutritious salad as a refreshing start to your day, packed with leafy greens, vegetables, and protein-rich eggs.

Feel free to customize the salad with your favorite ingredients or adapt it based on seasonal produce availability. This breakfast salad is not only delicious and satisfying but also a great way to incorporate vegetables and protein into your morning routine.

Chapter 3: Wholesome Lunches

- **Mediterranean Chickpea Salad**
- **Roasted Vegetable and Lentil Buddha Bowl**
- **Spinach and Feta Stuffed Bell Peppers**
- **Salmon and Avocado Nori Wraps**

Mediterranean Chickpea Salad

To prepare a Mediterranean Chickpea Salad, follow these simple steps:

Ingredients

- 2 cans (15 ounces each) chickpeas, drained and rinsed

- 1 English cucumber, diced

- 1 pint cherry tomatoes, halved

- 1/2 red onion, finely chopped

- 1/2 cup Kalamata olives, pitted and halved

- 1/4 cup fresh parsley, chopped

- 1/4 cup fresh mint leaves, chopped

- 1/3 cup crumbled feta cheese (optional)

- Juice of 1 lemon

- 3 tablespoons extra-virgin olive oil

- 2 cloves garlic, minced

- 1 teaspoon dried oregano

- Salt and black pepper to taste

Instructions

Prepare the Chickpeas: Drain and rinse the chickpeas under cold water. Pat them dry with a clean kitchen towel or paper towels.

Combine Ingredients: In a large mixing bowl, combine the chickpeas, diced cucumber, halved cherry tomatoes, chopped red onion, halved Kalamata olives, chopped parsley, and chopped mint leaves.

Make the Dressing: In a small bowl, whisk together the lemon juice, extra-virgin olive oil, minced garlic, dried oregano, salt, and black pepper to taste. Adjust the seasoning according to your preference.

Dress the Salad: Pour the dressing over the chickpea mixture in the large bowl. Gently toss until all the ingredients are evenly coated with the dressing.

Add Feta Cheese (Optional): If using crumbled feta cheese, sprinkle it over the salad and gently toss again to incorporate.

Chill and Serve: Cover the salad bowl with plastic wrap or transfer the salad to an airtight container. Refrigerate for at least 30 minutes to allow the flavors to meld together.

Serve: Before serving, give the salad a final toss. Taste and adjust the seasoning if necessary. Garnish with additional chopped herbs if desired.

Enjoy: Serve the Mediterranean Chickpea Salad as a refreshing side dish or a light and satisfying main course. It's perfect for picnics, potlucks, or as a nutritious addition to your meal.

This vibrant salad is packed with Mediterranean flavors, fiber, protein, and essential nutrients, making it both delicious and nourishing. Feel free to customize the salad by adding other ingredients such as diced bell peppers, artichoke hearts, or avocado slices according to your taste preferences.

<u>**Roasted Vegetable and Lentil Buddha Bowl**</u>

To prepare a Roasted Vegetable and Lentil Buddha Bowl, follow these steps:

Ingredients

1.For the Roasted Vegetables:

- 2 cups mixed vegetables (such as carrots, bell peppers, zucchini, broccoli, cauliflower), chopped into bite-sized pieces

- 2 tablespoons olive oil

- 1 teaspoon dried herbs (such as thyme, rosemary, or oregano)

- Salt and black pepper to taste

2.For the Lentils:

- 1 cup dried green or brown lentils

- 2 cups vegetable broth or water

- 1 bay leaf (optional)

- Salt to taste

3.For the Buddha Bowl Assembly:

- Cooked quinoa, rice, or couscous (optional base)

- Fresh spinach or mixed greens

- Avocado slices

- Cherry tomatoes, halved

- Sliced cucumber

- Hummus or tahini sauce for drizzling

- Lemon wedges for garnish

Instructions

1.Preheat the oven to 400°F (200°C).

2.Prepare the Roasted Vegetables:

- In a large mixing bowl, toss the chopped vegetables with olive oil, dried herbs, salt, and black pepper until evenly coated.

- Spread the vegetables in a single layer on a baking sheet lined with parchment paper.

- Roast in the preheated oven for 20-25 minutes or until the vegetables are tender and lightly browned, stirring halfway through cooking.

3.Cook the Lentils:

- Rinse the lentils under cold water and drain.

- In a medium saucepan, combine the lentils, vegetable broth or water, and bay leaf (if using).

- Bring the mixture to a boil over medium-high heat, then reduce the heat to low and simmer, covered, for 20-25 minutes or until the lentils are tender but not mushy.

- Drain any excess liquid from the lentils and discard the bay leaf. Season with salt to taste.

4.Assemble the Buddha Bowl:

- Start by placing a serving of cooked quinoa, rice, or couscous (if using) at the bottom of each bowl.

- Top with a handful of fresh spinach or mixed greens.

- Arrange the roasted vegetables, cooked lentils, avocado slices, cherry tomatoes, and sliced cucumber on top of the greens.

- Drizzle with hummus or tahini sauce for added flavor.

- Garnish with lemon wedges for squeezing over the bowl before eating.

5.Serve immediately and enjoy your wholesome and nourishing Roasted Vegetable and Lentil Buddha Bowl!

Feel free to customize your Buddha Bowl with your favorite vegetables, grains, proteins, and sauces according to your taste preferences and dietary needs. This versatile and satisfying meal is perfect for lunch or dinner and can be adapted to accommodate various dietary restrictions or preferences.

To prepare Spinach and Feta Stuffed Bell Peppers, follow these steps:

Ingredients

- 4 large bell peppers (any color)

- 2 cups fresh spinach, chopped

- 1 small onion, finely chopped

- 2 cloves garlic, minced

- 1 tablespoon olive oil

- 1 cup cooked quinoa or rice

- 1/2 cup crumbled feta cheese

- 1/4 cup grated Parmesan cheese (optional)

- 1 teaspoon dried oregano

- Salt and pepper to taste

- 1/4 cup chopped fresh parsley or basil for garnish

Instructions

1.Preheat the oven to 375°F (190°C). Grease a baking dish large enough to hold the bell peppers.

2.Prepare the Bell Peppers:

- Slice the tops off the bell peppers and remove the seeds and membranes from inside. Rinse the peppers under cold water and pat them dry with paper towels.

3.In a large skillet, heat the olive oil over medium heat. Add the chopped onion and minced garlic, and sauté until softened and fragrant, about 3-4 minutes.

4.Add the chopped spinach to the skillet and cook until wilted, stirring occasionally, about 2-3 minutes. Season with salt and pepper to taste.

5.In a large mixing bowl, combine the cooked quinoa or rice, sautéed spinach mixture, crumbled feta cheese, grated Parmesan cheese (if using), dried oregano, and chopped fresh parsley or basil. Mix well to combine.

6.Stuff the Bell Peppers:

- Divide the quinoa-spinach mixture evenly among the prepared bell peppers, packing the filling down gently with a spoon.

7.Place the stuffed bell peppers upright in the greased baking dish. If desired, sprinkle additional Parmesan cheese on top of each stuffed pepper.

8.Cover the baking dish with aluminum foil and bake in the preheated oven for 25-30 minutes, or until the peppers are tender and the filling is heated through.

9.Remove the foil during the last 10 minutes of baking to allow the cheese to melt and the tops of the peppers to brown slightly.

10.Once done, remove the stuffed bell peppers from the oven and let them cool for a few minutes before serving.

11.Serve the Spinach and Feta Stuffed Bell Peppers warm, garnished with additional chopped parsley or basil, if desired.

These Spinach and Feta Stuffed Bell Peppers make a delicious and nutritious meal or side dish. They are packed with flavor, protein, and vitamins, making them a satisfying and wholesome option for lunch or dinner. Enjoy!

Salmon and Avocado Nori Wraps

To prepare Salmon and Avocado Nori Wraps, follow these steps:

Ingredients

- 4 sheets of nori seaweed

- 2 (4-ounce) salmon fillets, cooked and flaked

- 1 ripe avocado, thinly sliced

- 1 small cucumber, julienned

- 1 small carrot, julienned

- 1/4 cup shredded red cabbage

- 2 tablespoons pickled ginger (optional)

- Soy sauce or tamari, for serving

- Wasabi paste, for serving (optional)

- Sesame seeds, for garnish (optional)

Instructions

1.Prepare the Ingredients:

- Cook the salmon fillets by grilling, baking, or pan-searing until fully cooked and flaky. Allow them to cool slightly before flaking them with a fork.

- Thinly slice the avocado and julienne the cucumber and carrot.
    - o
- Shred the red cabbage and prepare the pickled ginger if using.

2.Lay out a sheet of nori seaweed on a clean and dry surface, with the shiny side facing down.

3.Arrange the Fillings:

- Place a small portion of flaked salmon horizontally across the bottom third of the nori sheet, leaving a small border at the bottom.

- Layer slices of avocado, julienned cucumber, carrot, and shredded red cabbage over the salmon.

4.Roll the Nori Wrap:

- Starting from the bottom edge closest to you, tightly roll the nori sheet and filling upwards, using your fingers to keep the ingredients compact as you roll.

- Moisten the top border of the nori sheet with a little water to seal the roll.

5.Repeat the process with the remaining nori sheets and fillings.

6.Slice the Rolls:

- Use a sharp knife to slice each roll into bite-sized pieces, about 1 to 1.5 inches thick.

7.Serve and Garnish:

- Arrange the sliced nori wraps on a serving platter.

- Serve with soy sauce or tamari for dipping, and wasabi paste if desired.

- Garnish with sesame seeds for added flavor and presentation.

- Optionally, serve with pickled ginger on the side.

8.Enjoy your Salmon and Avocado Nori Wraps as a delicious and nutritious appetizer, snack, or light meal.

These wraps are not only tasty but also packed with healthy fats, protein, and essential nutrients from the salmon, avocado, and vegetables. They make a delightful addition to any meal or gathering, and their portable nature makes them perfect for on-the-go lunches or picnics.

Chapter 4: Nourishing Dinners

- **Lemon Garlic Herb Baked Chicken**
- **Spaghetti Squash Primavera**
- **Turmeric-Ginger Lentil Stew**
- **Seared Tuna with Sesame Broccoli**

Lemon Garlic Herb Baked Chicken

To prepare Lemon Garlic Herb Baked Chicken, follow these steps:

Ingredients:

- 4 boneless, skinless chicken breasts

- 4 cloves garlic, minced

- Zest of 1 lemon

- Juice of 1 lemon

- 2 tablespoons olive oil

- 1 teaspoon dried thyme

- 1 teaspoon dried rosemary

- 1 teaspoon dried oregano

- Salt and black pepper to taste

- Lemon slices for garnish

- Fresh herbs (such as parsley or thyme) for garnish

Instructions

1. Preheat the oven to 375°F (190°C). Grease a baking dish large enough to hold the chicken breasts.

2. In a small bowl, whisk together the minced garlic, lemon zest, lemon juice,

olive oil, dried thyme, dried rosemary, dried oregano, salt, and black pepper.

3. Place the chicken breasts in the prepared baking dish, arranging them in a single layer.

4. Pour the lemon garlic herb mixture over the chicken breasts, making sure they are evenly coated on all sides. You can use a brush or spoon to spread the mixture evenly.

5. If desired, you can add some lemon slices on top of the chicken breasts for extra flavor.

6. Bake the chicken in the preheated oven for 25-30 minutes, or until the chicken is cooked through and the juices run clear. The internal temperature of the chicken should reach 165°F (74°C).

7. Once done, remove the chicken from the oven and let it rest for a few minutes before serving.

8. Garnish the Lemon Garlic Herb Baked Chicken with fresh herbs, such as parsley or thyme, for added freshness and flavor.

9. Serve the chicken hot with your favorite side dishes, such as roasted vegetables, steamed rice, or mashed potatoes.

This Lemon Garlic Herb Baked Chicken recipe is simple to make and bursting with flavor. It's perfect for a quick and delicious weeknight dinner or a special meal with family and friends. Enjoy!

<u>Spaghetti Squash Primavera</u>

To prepare Spaghetti Squash Primavera, follow these steps:

Ingredients

- 1 medium spaghetti squash

- 2 tablespoons olive oil

- 3 cloves garlic, minced

- 1 small onion, finely chopped

- 1 bell pepper, diced

- 1 cup cherry tomatoes, halved

- 1 cup broccoli florets

- 1 cup sliced mushrooms

- 1 teaspoon dried Italian herbs (such as oregano, basil, thyme)

- Salt and black pepper to taste

- Grated Parmesan cheese (optional, for serving)

- Chopped fresh parsley or basil for garnish

Instructions:

1.Preheat the oven to 400°F (200°C). Line a baking sheet with parchment paper.

2.Cut the spaghetti squash in half lengthwise and scoop out the seeds and stringy pulp with a spoon.

3.Drizzle the cut sides of the spaghetti squash with olive oil and season with salt and black pepper.

4.Place the spaghetti squash halves cut-side down on the prepared baking sheet.

5.Bake in the preheated oven for 35-45 minutes, or until the squash is tender and the flesh easily shreds into strands with a fork. Cooking time may vary depending on the size of the squash.

6.While the spaghetti squash is baking, prepare the Primavera vegetables:

- In a large skillet, heat the remaining olive oil over medium heat. Add the minced garlic and chopped onion, and sauté until softened and fragrant, about 2-3 minutes.

- Add the diced bell pepper, halved cherry tomatoes, broccoli florets, and sliced mushrooms to the skillet. Cook, stirring occasionally, until the vegetables are tender-crisp, about 5-7 minutes.

- Season the vegetables with dried Italian herbs, salt, and black pepper to taste. Stir to combine and remove the skillet from heat.

7.Once the spaghetti squash is done baking, use a fork to scrape the flesh of the squash into strands, creating the "spaghetti."

8.Add the spaghetti squash strands to the skillet with the cooked vegetables. Toss everything together until well combined.

9. and adjust the seasoning if necessary.

10.Serve the Spaghetti Squash Primavera hot, garnished with grated Parmesan cheese (if using) and chopped fresh parsley or basil.

11.Enjoy this delicious and nutritious vegetarian meal as a light and satisfying lunch or dinner option!

This Spaghetti Squash Primavera recipe is not only flavorful and comforting but also low in carbohydrates and packed with vitamins, minerals, and fiber. It's a perfect dish for those looking to incorporate more vegetables into their diet or following a gluten-free or low-carb lifestyle.

Turmeric-Ginger Lentil Stew

To prepare Turmeric-Ginger Lentil Stew, follow these steps:

Ingredients

- 1 cup dried green or brown lentils, rinsed and drained

- 4 cups vegetable broth or water

- 2 tablespoons olive oil

- 1 onion, diced

- 3 cloves garlic, minced

- 1 tablespoon fresh ginger, grated

- 1 teaspoon ground turmeric

- 1 teaspoon ground cumin

- 1 teaspoon ground coriander

- 1/2 teaspoon ground cinnamon

- 1/4 teaspoon cayenne pepper (optional, for heat)

- 2 carrots, diced

- 2 celery stalks, diced

- 1 sweet potato, peeled and diced

- 1 can (14 ounces) diced tomatoes

- Salt and black pepper to taste

- Fresh cilantro or parsley for garnish (optional)

- Lemon wedges for serving (optional)

Instructions:

1. In a large pot or Dutch oven, heat the olive oil over medium heat.

2. Add the diced onion to the pot and sauté until it becomes translucent, about 3-4 minutes.

3. Stir in the minced garlic and grated ginger, and cook for another 1-2 minutes until fragrant.

4. Add the ground turmeric, ground cumin, ground coriander, ground cinnamon, and cayenne pepper (if using) to the pot. Stir well to coat the onions and garlic with the spices.

5. Add the diced carrots, diced celery, and diced sweet potato to the pot. Stir to combine with the onion and spice mixture.

6. Pour in the rinsed and drained lentils and diced tomatoes (with their juices) into the pot.

7. Add the vegetable broth or water to the pot, ensuring that the ingredients are fully submerged.

8. Bring the stew to a boil, then reduce the heat to low and let it simmer, partially covered, for about 25-30 minutes, or until the lentils and vegetables are tender.

9. Season the stew with salt and black pepper to taste. Adjust the seasoning if necessary.

10. Serve the Turmeric-Ginger Lentil Stew hot, garnished with fresh cilantro or parsley if desired, and with lemon wedges on the side for squeezing over the stew before eating.

11. Enjoy this comforting and nutritious stew as a hearty meal on its own or serve it with crusty bread or rice for a complete and satisfying dinner.

This Turmeric-Ginger Lentil Stew is not only delicious and aromatic but also loaded with plant-based protein, fiber, and essential nutrients. It's a perfect dish to warm you up on chilly days and support your overall health and well-being.

<u>Seared Tuna with Sesame Broccoli</u>

To prepare Seared Tuna with Sesame Broccoli, follow these steps:

Ingredients

- For the Seared Tuna:

- 2 tuna steaks, about 6 ounces each

- 2 tablespoons soy sauce

- 1 tablespoon sesame oil

- 1 tablespoon lime juice

- 1 tablespoon honey or maple syrup

- 2 cloves garlic, minced

- 1 teaspoon grated ginger

- 1 tablespoon sesame seeds

- Salt and pepper to taste

- 2 tablespoons olive oil (for searing)

For the Sesame Broccoli

- 1 head broccoli, cut into florets

- 2 tablespoons soy sauce

- 1 tablespoon sesame oil

- 1 tablespoon sesame seeds

- 2 cloves garlic, minced

- Salt and pepper to taste

Instructions

1.Prepare the Seared Tuna:

- In a shallow dish, combine the soy sauce, sesame oil, lime juice, honey or maple syrup, minced garlic, grated ginger, sesame seeds, salt, and pepper. Mix well to make the marinade.

- Place the tuna steaks in the marinade, turning to coat both sides evenly. Cover and refrigerate for at least 30 minutes to allow the flavors to infuse.

2.Prepare the Sesame Broccoli:

- In a large bowl, toss the broccoli florets with soy sauce, sesame oil, minced garlic, sesame seeds, salt, and pepper until well coated.

3.Heat a skillet or frying pan over medium-high heat. Add the olive oil for searing.

4.Once the pan is hot, remove the tuna steaks from the marinade, shaking off any excess liquid. Reserve the marinade for later use.

5.Place the tuna steaks in the skillet and sear for about 1-2 minutes on each side, or until desired doneness. For medium-rare, aim for a slightly pink center.

6.While the tuna is searing, preheat the oven to 400°F (200°C).

7.Transfer the seared tuna to a baking dish and brush with the reserved marinade.

8.Roast the tuna in the preheated oven for 5-7 minutes for medium-rare, or longer if desired.

9.While the tuna is roasting, spread the seasoned broccoli florets evenly on a baking sheet lined with parchment paper.

10.Roast the broccoli in the preheated oven for 15-20 minutes, or until tender and slightly crispy around the edges.

11.Once the tuna and broccoli are done, remove them from the oven.

12.Serve the Seared Tuna with Sesame Broccoli hot, garnished with additional sesame seeds if desired.

13.Enjoy this flavorful and nutritious dish as a satisfying main course for lunch or dinner.

This Seared Tuna with Sesame Broccoli recipe offers a delightful combination of flavors and textures, making it a perfect option for seafood lovers seeking a healthy and delicious meal. Adjust the cooking times according to your preferred level of doneness for the tuna.

Chapter 5: Snacks and Small Bites

- **Crunchy Edamame Snack**
- **Almond Butter and Banana Rice Cakes**
- **Greek Yogurt Parfait with Honey and Berries**
- **Roasted Beet Hummus with Veggie Sticks**

Crunchy Edamame Snack

To prepare Crunchy Edamame Snack, follow these steps:

Ingredients:

- 2 cups frozen edamame (unshelled)

- 1 tablespoon olive oil or avocado oil

- 1 tablespoon soy sauce or tamari (for a gluten-free option)

- 1 teaspoon garlic powder

- 1 teaspoon onion powder

- 1/2 teaspoon smoked paprika (optional)

- Salt to taste

Instructions

1. Preheat the oven to 400°F (200°C). Line a baking sheet with parchment paper or lightly grease it with oil to prevent sticking.

2. Thaw the frozen edamame by rinsing them under cold water in a colander. Drain well and pat dry with paper towels to remove excess moisture.

3. In a mixing bowl, combine the thawed edamame with olive oil, soy sauce or tamari, garlic powder, onion powder, smoked paprika (if using), and salt to taste. Toss well until the edamame are evenly coated with the seasonings.

4. Spread the seasoned edamame in a single layer on the prepared baking sheet.

5. Roast the edamame in the preheated oven for 15-20 minutes, stirring halfway through, or until they are crispy and lightly golden brown.

6. Once done, remove the baking sheet from the oven and let the crunchy edamame cool slightly before serving.

7. Serve the Crunchy Edamame Snack as a delicious and nutritious appetizer, side dish, or crunchy snack on its own.

8. Store any leftovers in an airtight container at room temperature for up to 2-3 days. Note that the crunchiness may diminish over time, but the flavor will remain delicious.

This Crunchy Edamame Snack is not only tasty but also packed with protein, fiber, and essential nutrients. Enjoy it as a guilt-free snack option or a flavorful addition to your favorite salads or Buddha bowls.

<u>**Almond Butter and Banana Rice Cakes**</u>

To prepare Almond Butter and Banana Rice Cakes, follow these simple steps:

Ingredients

- 4 rice cakes (choose your favorite variety)

- 1 ripe banana, thinly sliced

- 4 tablespoons almond butter (or any nut or seed butter of your choice)

- Honey or maple syrup, for drizzling (optional)

- Cinnamon, for sprinkling (optional)

- Chia seeds, hemp seeds, or sliced almonds, for topping (optional)

Instructions

1. Arrange the rice cakes on a clean and dry surface, such as a plate or cutting board.

2. Spread about 1 tablespoon of almond butter evenly over each rice cake, covering the surface.

3. Place thinly sliced banana rounds on top of the almond butter layer, arranging them in a single layer.

4. Drizzle honey or maple syrup over the banana slices for added sweetness, if desired.

5. Sprinkle a pinch of cinnamon over the banana slices for extra flavor, if desired.

6. Optionally, add a sprinkle of chia seeds, hemp seeds, or sliced almonds on top of the banana slices for added texture and nutrition.

7. Repeat the process for the remaining rice cakes.

8. Serve the Almond Butter and Banana Rice Cakes immediately as a delicious and nutritious snack or light breakfast option.

This recipe is versatile and can be customized to suit your taste preferences. Feel free to experiment with different nut or seed butters, fruit toppings, and additional toppings such as shredded coconut or dark chocolate chips. Enjoy the combination of creamy almond butter, sweet banana, and crunchy rice cakes for a satisfying and wholesome treat!

<u>**Greek Yogurt Parfait with Honey and Berries**</u>

To prepare a Greek Yogurt Parfait with Honey and Berries, follow these simple steps:

Ingredients

- 1 cup Greek yogurt (plain or vanilla flavored)

- 2 tablespoons honey (or maple syrup, if preferred)

- 1 cup mixed berries (such as strawberries, blueberries, raspberries)

- Granola or muesli for layering

- Optional toppings: sliced almonds, shredded coconut, chia seeds

Instructions

1. Wash and prepare the mixed berries by slicing any larger fruits, if necessary.

2. In a small bowl, mix the Greek yogurt with honey until well combined. Adjust the amount of honey to suit your desired level of sweetness.

3. Start layering the parfait in serving glasses or bowls. Begin with a spoonful of Greek yogurt at the bottom of each glass.

4. Add a layer of mixed berries on top of the yogurt.

5. Sprinkle a layer of granola or muesli over the berries.

6. Repeat the layers by adding more yogurt, berries, and granola until the glasses are filled or you have reached your desired amount.

7. Finish off the parfait with a final drizzle of honey on top for added sweetness, if desired.

8. Optionally, sprinkle sliced almonds, shredded coconut, or chia seeds over the top for extra flavor and texture.

9. Repeat the layering process for each serving glass or bowl until all ingredients are used.

10. Serve the Greek Yogurt Parfait with Honey and Berries immediately as a nutritious and refreshing breakfast, snack, or dessert option.

This simple and versatile parfait recipe is customizable based on your preferences and the ingredients you have on hand. Feel free to experiment with different types of yogurt, fruits, sweeteners, and toppings to create your perfect parfait combination. Enjoy the creamy yogurt, sweet berries, and crunchy granola in every delightful spoonful!

Roasted Beet Hummus with Veggie Sticks

To prepare Roasted Beet Hummus with Veggie Sticks, follow these steps:

Ingredients

- For the Roasted Beet Hummus:

- 1 medium-sized beet, washed and trimmed

- 1 can (15 ounces) chickpeas, drained and rinsed

- 2 cloves garlic, minced

- 1/4 cup tahini (sesame paste)

- 3 tablespoons lemon juice (about 1 large lemon)

- 2 tablespoons olive oil

- 1/2 teaspoon ground cumin

- Salt and pepper to taste

- Water (as needed for consistency)

For Serving:

- Assorted vegetable sticks (carrots, cucumbers, bell peppers, celery, etc.)

- Pita bread or whole grain crackers (optional)

Instructions:

1. Preheat the oven to 400°F (200°C).

2. Wrap the washed and trimmed beet in aluminum foil and place it on a baking sheet. Roast the beet in the preheated oven for about 45-60 minutes, or until tender when pierced with a fork.

3. Once the beet is roasted and cooled, peel off the skin and cut it into chunks.

4. In a food processor or blender, combine the roasted beet chunks, drained and rinsed chickpeas, minced garlic, tahini, lemon juice, olive oil, ground cumin, salt, and pepper.

5. Blend the ingredients until smooth and creamy, scraping down the sides of the bowl or blender as needed. If the hummus is too thick, you can add water, 1 tablespoon at a time, until you reach your desired consistency.

6. Taste the hummus and adjust the seasoning if necessary, adding more salt, pepper, or lemon juice according to your preference.

7. Once the hummus is smooth and well blended, transfer it to a serving bowl.

8. Prepare the vegetable sticks by washing and cutting them into bite-sized pieces. Arrange them on a platter alongside the hummus.

9. Optionally, serve the roasted beet hummus with pita bread or whole grain crackers for dipping.

10.Garnish the hummus with a drizzle of olive oil, a sprinkle of sesame seeds, or fresh herbs if desired.

11.Serve the Roasted Beet Hummus with Veggie Sticks as a colorful and nutritious appetizer, snack, or party dip.

This vibrant and flavorful hummus is not only delicious but also packed with nutrients and antioxidants from the roasted beet. It's a healthy and visually appealing option for entertaining guests or enjoying a wholesome snack any time of the day.

Chapter 6: Sweet Treats for Balance

- **Dark Chocolate Avocado Mousse**
- **Coconut Chia Seed Pudding**
- **Berry and Almond Flour Crisp**
- **Banana-Oatmeal Cookies with Walnuts**

Dark Chocolate Avocado Mousse

To prepare Dark Chocolate Avocado Mousse, follow these steps:

Ingredients:

- 2 ripe avocados, peeled and pitted

- 1/4 cup unsweetened cocoa powder

- 1/4 cup maple syrup or honey (adjust to taste)

- 1 teaspoon vanilla extract

- Pinch of salt

- 1/4 cup almond milk or any milk of your choice (optional, for desired consistency)

- Dark chocolate shavings or cocoa nibs for garnish (optional)

- Fresh berries for garnish (optional)

Instructions

1. In a food processor or blender, combine the ripe avocados, unsweetened cocoa powder, maple syrup or honey, vanilla extract, and a pinch of salt.

2. Blend the ingredients until smooth and creamy, scraping down the sides of the bowl or blender as needed to ensure everything is well combined.

3. Taste the mousse and adjust the sweetness by adding more maple syrup or honey if desired.

4. If the mousse is too thick, add almond milk or any milk of your choice, 1 tablespoon at a time, until you reach your desired consistency. Blend again until smooth.

5. Once the mousse reaches the desired consistency and taste, transfer it to serving bowls or glasses.

6. Cover the bowls or glasses with plastic wrap and refrigerate the mousse for at least 30 minutes to chill and firm up.

7. Before serving, garnish the Dark Chocolate Avocado Mousse with dark chocolate shavings, cocoa nibs, or fresh berries for added flavor and presentation.

8. Serve the mousse chilled and enjoy its rich and creamy texture.

This Dark Chocolate Avocado Mousse is a healthier alternative to traditional mousse recipes, as it's made with nutritious avocado and natural sweeteners. It's also vegan and gluten-free, making it suitable for various dietary preferences. Enjoy this decadent treat as a delicious dessert or snack that's both satisfying and guilt-free!

Coconut Chia Seed Pudding

To prepare Coconut Chia Seed Pudding, follow these steps:

Ingredients:

- 1/4 cup chia seeds

- 1 cup coconut milk (canned or homemade)

- 1 tablespoon maple syrup or honey (optional, adjust to taste)

- 1/2 teaspoon vanilla extract

- Fresh fruit, such as berries or sliced mango, for topping (optional)

- Toasted coconut flakes, for garnish (optional)

Instructions

1. In a mixing bowl or jar, combine the chia seeds, coconut milk, maple syrup or honey (if using), and vanilla extract.

2. Whisk the ingredients together until well combined. Make sure the chia seeds are evenly distributed throughout the mixture.

3. Cover the bowl or jar and refrigerate the mixture for at least 2-3 hours, or preferably overnight. This allows the chia seeds to absorb the liquid and thicken into a pudding-like consistency.

4. After the pudding has set, give it a good stir to ensure that any chia seeds stuck to the bottom are incorporated into the pudding.

5. Taste the pudding and adjust the sweetness if necessary by adding more maple syrup or honey.

6. Serve the Coconut Chia Seed Pudding chilled, either on its own or layered with fresh fruit, such as berries or sliced mango.

7. Optionally, garnish the pudding with toasted coconut flakes for added texture and flavor.

8. Enjoy this delicious and nutritious pudding as a healthy breakfast, snack, or dessert option.

This Coconut Chia Seed Pudding is not only tasty but also packed with fiber, omega-3 fatty acids, and essential nutrients. It's also dairy-free, vegan, and gluten-free, making it suitable for a variety of dietary preferences. Experiment with different toppings and flavor variations to customize the pudding to your liking.

<u>**Berry and Almond Flour Crisp**</u>

To prepare a Berry and Almond Flour Crisp, follow these steps:

Ingredients:

For the Berry Filling:

- 4 cups mixed berries (such as strawberries, blueberries, raspberries, blackberries)

- 1/4 cup granulated sugar (adjust to taste)

- 2 tablespoons cornstarch

- 1 tablespoon lemon juice

- Zest of 1 lemon

For the Almond Flour Crisp Topping:

- 1 cup almond flour

- 1/2 cup old-fashioned rolled oats

- 1/4 cup packed brown sugar

- 1/4 teaspoon salt

- 1/2 teaspoon ground cinnamon

- 1/4 cup cold unsalted butter, cut into small pieces

- 1/4 cup sliced almonds (optional, for extra crunch)

Instructions:

1. Preheat the oven to 350°F (175°C). Grease a 9x9 inch baking dish or a similar-sized baking dish with butter or non-stick cooking spray.

2. In a large mixing bowl, combine the mixed berries, granulated sugar, cornstarch, lemon juice, and lemon zest.

Toss until the berries are evenly coated with the sugar and cornstarch mixture.

3. Transfer the berry mixture to the prepared baking dish, spreading it out evenly.

4. In a separate mixing bowl, combine the almond flour, rolled oats, brown sugar, salt, and ground cinnamon. Stir until well combined.

5. Add the cold butter pieces to the almond flour mixture. Using your fingers or a pastry cutter, work the butter into the dry ingredients until the mixture resembles coarse crumbs and the butter is evenly distributed.

6. If using sliced almonds, gently fold them into the crisp topping mixture.

7. Sprinkle the almond flour crisp topping evenly over the berry mixture in the baking dish.

8. Place the baking dish in the preheated oven and bake for 35-40 minutes, or until the berry filling is bubbly and the crisp topping is golden brown and crispy.

9. Once done, remove the Berry and Almond Flour Crisp from the oven and let it cool for a few minutes before serving.

10. Serve the crisp warm, optionally topped with a scoop of vanilla ice cream or a dollop of whipped cream for an extra treat.

11. Enjoy this delightful Berry and Almond Flour Crisp as a comforting dessert, perfect for sharing with family and friends!

Feel free to customize the crisp by using your favorite combination of berries or adjusting the sweetness level according to your taste preferences. This wholesome

<u>Banana-Oatmeal Cookies with Walnuts</u>

To prepare Banana-Oatmeal Cookies with Walnuts, follow these steps:

Ingredients

- 2 ripe bananas, mashed

- 1 1/2 cups rolled oats

- 1/2 cup chopped walnuts

- 1/4 cup maple syrup or honey

- 1/4 cup melted coconut oil or melted butter

- 1 teaspoon vanilla extract

- 1/2 teaspoon ground cinnamon

- 1/4 teaspoon salt

- Optional add-ins: chocolate chips, raisins, dried cranberries

Instructions:

1. Preheat the oven to 350°F (175°C). Line a baking sheet with parchment paper or lightly grease it with cooking spray.

2. In a large mixing bowl, mash the ripe bananas with a fork until smooth.

3. Add the rolled oats, chopped walnuts, maple syrup or honey, melted coconut oil or melted butter, vanilla extract, ground cinnamon, and salt to the bowl with the mashed bananas.

4. Stir all the ingredients together until well combined and the mixture forms a thick dough. If the dough seems too dry, you can add a splash of milk to moisten it slightly.

5. If desired, fold in any optional add-ins such as chocolate chips, raisins, or dried cranberries into the cookie dough.

6. Using a spoon or cookie scoop, drop spoonfuls of the cookie dough onto the prepared baking sheet, spacing them a few inches apart.

7. Use your fingers or the back of a spoon to gently flatten each cookie dough mound into a cookie shape.

8. Bake the cookies in the preheated oven for 12-15 minutes, or until the cookies are golden brown around the edges and set in the center.

9. Once done, remove the baking sheet from the oven and let the cookies cool on the baking sheet for a few minutes before transferring them to a wire rack to cool completely.

10. Allow the Banana-Oatmeal Cookies with Walnuts to cool completely before serving or storing in an airtight container.

11. Enjoy these delicious and wholesome cookies as a healthy snack or dessert option!

These Banana-Oatmeal Cookies with Walnuts are not only easy to make but also nutritious and satisfying. They're perfect for using up ripe bananas and make a great grab-and-go snack for busy days. Feel free to customize the recipe by adding your favorite mix-ins or adjusting the sweetness level to suit your taste preferences.

Chapter 7: Beverages for Fertility Wellness

- **Green Goddess Smoothie**
- **Turmeric Golden Milk**
- **Berry Blast Infused Water**
- **Fertility Herbal Tea Blend**

Green Goddess Smoothie

To prepare a Green Goddess Smoothie, follow these steps:

Ingredients:

- 1 ripe banana, peeled and sliced

- 1/2 cup frozen mango chunks

- 1/2 cup fresh spinach leaves (or kale)

- 1/4 cup fresh cilantro leaves (or parsley)

- 1/4 cup fresh mint leaves

- 1/2 avocado, peeled and pitted

- 1 cup unsweetened almond milk (or any milk of your choice)

- 1 tablespoon honey or maple syrup (optional, for added sweetness)

- Juice of 1/2 lime or lemon

- Ice cubes (optional, for a colder smoothie)

Instructions

1. Place all the ingredients in a blender in the order listed: sliced banana, frozen mango chunks, fresh spinach leaves, cilantro leaves, mint leaves, avocado, almond milk, honey or maple syrup (if using), and lime or lemon juice.

2. If desired, add a handful of ice cubes to the blender to make the smoothie colder.

3. Blend the ingredients on high speed until smooth and creamy, scraping down the sides of the blender as needed to ensure all ingredients are well incorporated.

4. Taste the smoothie and adjust the sweetness or acidity by adding more honey, maple syrup, lime juice, or lemon juice as needed.

5. Once the desired consistency and flavor are achieved, pour the Green Goddess Smoothie into glasses.

6. Garnish the smoothie with additional mint leaves or a slice of lime or lemon for presentation, if desired.

7. Serve the Green Goddess Smoothie immediately and enjoy its refreshing and nutritious flavors!

This Green Goddess Smoothie is packed with vitamins, minerals, and antioxidants from the fruits and vegetables, making it a perfect option for a healthy breakfast, snack, or post-workout refresher. Feel free to customize the smoothie by adding protein powder, flaxseeds, chia seeds, or other favorite ingredients to boost its nutritional content.

<u>**Turmeric Golden Milk**</u>

To prepare Turmeric Golden Milk, follow these steps:

Ingredients

- 2 cups milk (dairy or plant-based such as almond, coconut, or soy milk)

- 1 teaspoon ground turmeric

- 1/2 teaspoon ground cinnamon

- 1/4 teaspoon ground ginger (or 1/2 teaspoon freshly grated ginger)

- 1 tablespoon honey or maple syrup (adjust to taste)

- 1/2 teaspoon vanilla extract (optional)

- Pinch of ground black pepper (helps with turmeric absorption)

- Pinch of ground nutmeg (optional)

- Pinch of ground cardamom (optional)

Instructions

1. In a small saucepan, heat the milk over medium-low heat until it begins to steam, but not boil. Stir occasionally to prevent scalding.

2. Add the ground turmeric, ground cinnamon, ground ginger, honey or maple syrup, vanilla extract (if using), and a pinch of black pepper to the saucepan.

3. Whisk the ingredients together until well combined and the spices are fully dissolved into the milk.

4. Continue to heat the mixture for another 2-3 minutes, stirring occasionally, until it is hot and fragrant.

5. Taste the golden milk and adjust the sweetness or spiciness by adding more honey, maple syrup, or spices as desired.

6. Once the golden milk is heated through and infused with the flavors of the spices, remove the saucepan from the heat.

7. Strain the golden milk through a fine-mesh sieve or tea strainer into serving mugs to remove any spice particles of sediment.

8. Sprinkle a pinch of ground nutmeg and ground cardamom over the top of each mug for extra flavor and aroma, if desired.

9. Serve the Turmeric Golden Milk warm and enjoy its soothing and comforting qualities.

This Turmeric Golden Milk is not only delicious but also packed with anti-inflammatory and antioxidant properties thanks to the turmeric and other spices. It's a cozy and nourishing drink that's perfect for sipping in the evening or anytime you need a warming and comforting beverage. Adjust the ingredients to suit your taste preferences and enjoy the health benefits of this golden elixir.

<u>**Berry Blast Infused Water**</u>

To prepare Berry Blast Infused Water, follow these steps:

Ingredients:

- 1 cup mixed berries (such as strawberries, blueberries, raspberries, blackberries)

- 6-8 cups water (filtered or spring water)

- Ice cubes (optional, for serving)

- Fresh mint leaves (optional, for garnish)

Instructions:

1. Wash the mixed berries thoroughly under cold running water to remove any dirt or debris. Pat them dry with a paper towel.

2. Slice larger berries such as strawberries into halves or quarters to release more flavor.

3. In a large pitcher, add the mixed berries to the bottom.

4. Fill the pitcher with 6-8 cups of water, depending on the size of the pitcher and your preference for the strength of the infused flavor.

5. Use a spoon or a muddler to gently press on the berries to release their juices and flavors into the water.

6. Cover the pitcher and refrigerate the Berry Blast Infused Water for at least 2-4 hours, or overnight for a stronger flavor infusion.

7. When ready to serve, you can add ice cubes to the individual glasses or directly to the pitcher to make the infused water colder and more refreshing.

8. Optionally, garnish each glass with fresh mint leaves for a pop of color and extra freshness.

9. Stir the infused water before serving to redistribute the flavors evenly.

10.Serve the Berry Blast Infused Water chilled and enjoy its refreshing and fruity taste.

This Berry Blast Infused Water is a delicious and hydrating way to enjoy the natural flavors of mixed berries while staying hydrated throughout the day. Feel free to customize the recipe by adding other fruits, herbs, or citrus slices for different flavor combinations. It's a healthy and refreshing beverage option for any occasion.

<u>**Fertility Herbal Tea Blend**</u>

Creating a fertility herbal tea blend can be a holistic approach to support reproductive health. Here's a basic recipe for a fertility herbal tea blend:

Ingredients

Raspberry Leaf: Raspberry leaf is known for its toning effect on the uterus and can help prepare the uterus for pregnancy.

Red Clover Blossoms: Red clover blossoms are rich in vitamins and minerals that support overall reproductive health. They are believed to help balance hormones and support fertility.

Nettle Leaf: Nettle leaf is a nutrient-rich herb that contains vitamins and minerals essential for reproductive health, including iron and calcium.

Dong Quai (Angelica sinensis): Dong Quai is a traditional Chinese herb known for its ability to regulate menstrual cycles and support hormone balance. It's often used in herbal blends for women's reproductive health.

Vitex (Chaste Tree Berry): Vitex is an herb commonly used to support hormone balance and regulate menstrual cycles, which can be beneficial for women trying to conceive.

Instructions:

1. Combine equal parts of each herb in a clean glass jar or container. You can start with 1 tablespoon of each herb for a small batch.

2. Mix the herbs thoroughly to create your fertility herbal tea blend.

3. Store the herbal blend in an airtight container away from direct sunlight and heat.

4. To prepare the tea, add 1-2 teaspoons of the herbal blend to a tea infuser for teapot.

5. Pour hot water over the herbs and let them steep for 5-10 minutes, depending on your preference for strength.

6.

7. Strain the tea and discard the herbs.

8. You can sweeten the tea with honey or add lemon juice if desired.

9. Enjoy the fertility herbal tea blend 1-2 times per day, preferably during the follicular phase of the menstrual cycle (from the end of menstruation to ovulation).

Note: It's essential to consult with a healthcare professional before incorporating any herbal remedies, including fertility herbal tea blends, especially if you have any underlying health conditions or are taking medications. While herbs can offer support for fertility, they should be used as part of a comprehensive approach to reproductive health and not as a standalone treatment.

Chapter 8: Meal Planning and Preparing for Fertility Success

- **Tips for Meal Prepping and Planning**
- **Incorporating Fertility-Boosting Ingredients Into Your Diet**
- **Fertility-Friendly Ingredient Substitutions**
- **Building a Supportive Environment for Your Fertility Journey**

Tips for Meal Prepping and Planning

Meal planning and preparation play crucial roles in supporting fertility success by providing the body with essential nutrients, supporting hormonal balance, and maintaining overall health. Here's a guide to meal planning and preparing for fertility success:

Focus on Whole Foods:

- Base your meals around whole, nutrient-dense foods such as fruits, vegetables, whole grains, lean proteins, healthy fats, and legumes.

- Choose organic and locally sourced foods when possible to reduce exposure to pesticides and chemicals.

Include Fertility-Boosting Foods:

- Incorporate foods rich in antioxidants, vitamins, and minerals that support fertility, such as leafy greens, berries, nuts, seeds, fatty fish (rich in omega-3 fatty acids), and legumes.

- Include foods high in folate, iron, zinc, vitamin D, vitamin C, and B vitamins, which are essential for reproductive health.

Prioritize Protein:

- Ensure you're getting an adequate amount of protein from sources such as lean meats, poultry, fish, eggs, dairy products, tofu, tempeh, beans, and lentils.

- Protein is essential for hormone production, egg quality, and overall reproductive health.

Choose Healthy Fats:

- Incorporate healthy fats from sources such as avocados, nuts, seeds, olive oil, coconut oil, and fatty fish.

- Omega-3 fatty acids, in particular, are beneficial for hormone balance and reproductive function.

Limit Processed Foods and Added Sugars:

- Minimize consumption of processed foods, refined carbohydrates, and added sugars, which can negatively impact hormonal balance and fertility.

- Opt for whole food alternatives whenever possible.

Stay Hydrated:

- Drink plenty of water throughout the day to stay hydrated and support overall health and fertility.

- Herbal teas, infused water, and coconut water are also refreshing options.

Incorporate Fertility-Boosting Herbs and Spices:

- Certain herbs and spices such as ginger, turmeric, cinnamon, and maca root may support hormonal balance and reproductive health. Incorporate them into your meals and beverages as desired.

Practice Portion Control:

- Pay attention to portion sizes to avoid overeating and maintain a healthy weight, which is important for fertility.

- Aim for balanced meals that include a variety of nutrients from different food groups.

Meal Prep and Planning:

- Plan your meals and snacks ahead of time to ensure you have nutritious options readily available.

- Spend time on weekends or during free time preparing meals, chopping vegetables, and pre-cooking ingredients to streamline the cooking process during the week.

Seek Professional Guidance:

- Consult with a registered dietitian or nutritionist specializing in fertility and reproductive health for personalized dietary recommendations and guidance.

Incorporating fertility-boosting ingredients into your diet can support reproductive health and optimize your chances of conception. Here are some key fertility-boosting ingredients and how to incorporate them into your meals:

Leafy Greens:

- Leafy greens such as spinach, kale, Swiss chard, and collard greens are rich in folate, iron, and other essential nutrients that support reproductive health.

- Add spinach to omelette, smoothies, salads, and pasta dishes.

- Sauté kale with garlic and olive oil as a side dish or add it to soups and stews.

Berries:

- Berries like strawberries, blueberries, raspberries, and blackberries are high in antioxidants and vitamin C, which may help improve egg quality and overall fertility.

- Enjoy berries as a topping for yogurt, oatmeal, or cereal.

- Blend berries into smoothies or add them to salads for a burst of flavor and nutrients.

Fatty Fish:

- Fatty fish such as salmon, mackerel, sardines, and trout are rich in omega-3 fatty acids, which support hormone regulation and reproductive health.

- Grill or bake salmon fillets and serve with roasted vegetables.

- Add canned sardines to salads or enjoy them on whole grain toast.

Nuts and Seeds:

- Nuts and seeds like almonds, walnuts, flaxseeds, and chia seeds are excellent sources of healthy fats, protein, and fiber that support hormonal balance and reproductive health.

- Snack on a handful of mixed nuts and seeds for a nutritious pick-me-up.

- Sprinkle ground flaxseeds or chia seeds over yogurt, oatmeal, or smoothie bowls.

Whole Grains:

- Whole grains such as quinoa, brown rice, oats, and barley are rich in fiber, B vitamins, and minerals that support fertility and reproductive health.

- Cook quinoa and use it as a base for grain bowls or salads.

- Enjoy oatmeal topped with fresh fruit, nuts, and seeds for breakfast.

Legumes:

- Legumes such as lentils, chickpeas, black beans, and kidney beans are excellent sources of plant-based protein, fiber, and folate, which support hormonal balance and fertility.

- Make homemade hummus using chickpeas and enjoy it as a dip or spread.

- Add cooked lentils or beans to soups, salads, and stir-fries for extra protein and fiber.

Avocado:

- Avocado is rich in healthy monounsaturated fats, vitamins E and C, and potassium, which support hormonal balance and reproductive health.

- Mash avocado and spread it on whole grain toast or use it as a creamy dressing for salads.

- Add sliced avocado to sandwiches, wraps, and omelets for extra flavor and nutrients.

Incorporating these fertility-boosting ingredients into your diet can help support reproductive health and optimize fertility. Aim for a balanced and varied diet that includes a variety of nutrient-dense foods to nourish your body and enhance your chances of conception.

You may enhance your chances of conception and maintain reproductive health by including foods high in fertility in your diet. You may replace the following ingredients in your meals to increase fertility:

Complete Grains: Replace processed grains like white bread and rice with healthy grains like barley, brown rice, quinoa, and whole wheat pasta or bread. Fiber, vitamins, minerals, and antioxidants included in whole grains help maintain hormonal balance and general health.

Good Fats: Healthy fats from sources like avocados, almonds, seeds, and olive oil may take the role of trans and saturated fats. Essential fatty acids, which are necessary for hormone synthesis and reproductive health, are provided by these fats.

Trim Proteins: Select lean protein sources over processed meats and fatty meat cuts, such as fish, chicken, tofu, tempeh, beans, and lentils.

Fertility depends on minerals like iron, zinc, and amino acids, all of which are abundant in lean proteins.

Greens with leaves: Include leafy greens in your meals, such as collard greens, Swiss chard, spinach, and kale. Rich in vitamins, minerals, and folate, leafy greens promote reproductive health and lower the incidence of birth abnormalities.

Berries: Include berries in your diet, such as raspberries, blackberries, blueberries, and strawberries. Berries are rich in fiber, vitamins, and antioxidants that promote the quality of sperm and eggs while reducing inflammation and oxidative stress.

Bright Vegetables: Incorporate a range of vibrant veggies into your meals, such as tomatoes, bell peppers, carrots, and sweet potatoes. A variety of vitamins, minerals, and antioxidants found in these veggies boost immunological and reproductive health.

Plant-Based Proteins: Include plant-based protein sources in your diet, such as edamame, lentils, beans, and chickpeas. High in fiber, phytonutrients, and antioxidants, plant-based proteins have the potential to enhance fertility and balance hormones.

Nutritious Spices and Herbs: When cooking, use herbs and spices such as garlic, ginger, turmeric, and cinnamon. The anti-inflammatory and antioxidant qualities of these herbs and spices promote hormone balance and reproductive health.

Glycemic-Reduced Sweeteners: Instead of processed sugars, use low-glycemic sweeteners like stevia, honey, and maple syrup. Blood sugar swings brought on by high-glycemic meals may have a deleterious effect on fertility.

The Fatty Acids Omega-3: Consume foods high in omega-3 fatty acids, such as walnuts, flaxseeds, chia seeds, and fatty fish (salmon, mackerel, and sardines). Healthy egg and sperm development, inflammation reduction, and hormone synthesis are all supported by omega-3 fatty acids.

These fertility-friendly ingredient replacements allow you to prepare wholesome, well-balanced meals that enhance reproductive health and help you reach your goals of conception. Remember that for individualized nutritional advice based on your unique requirements and medical circumstances, speak with a healthcare professional or a licensed dietitian.

Building a Supportive Environment for Your Fertility Journey

Building a supportive environment for your fertility journey involves creating a holistic approach that encompasses various aspects of your life, including physical, emotional, and environmental factors. Here are some strategies to help create a supportive environment for your fertility journey:

Nutritious Diet: Focus on consuming a balanced and nutritious diet rich in fruits, vegetables, whole grains, lean proteins, healthy fats, and fertility-boosting foods. Incorporate foods that support reproductive health and hormonal balance.

Regular Exercise: Engage in regular physical activity to help manage stress, maintain a healthy weight, and support overall well-being. Choose activities you enjoy, such as walking, swimming, yoga, or cycling.

Manage Stress: Practice stress-reducing techniques such as meditation, deep breathing exercises, mindfulness, yoga, or tai chi to help reduce stress levels and promote relaxation. Chronic stress can negatively impact fertility, so finding healthy ways to manage stress is essential.

Seek Emotional Support: Share your feelings and experiences with trusted friends, family members, or a support group who can offer empathy, understanding, and encouragement. Consider seeking professional counseling or therapy to help cope with the emotional challenges of infertility.

Maintain a Positive Outlook: Stay hopeful and optimistic about your fertility journey, focusing on the things within your control and acknowledging that setbacks are a normal part of the process. Practice gratitude and celebrate small victories along the way.

Educate Yourself: Educate yourself about fertility, reproductive health, and treatment options available to you. Ask questions, seek reliable information from reputable sources, and consider consulting with fertility specialists or healthcare providers to explore your options.

Create a Relaxing Environment: Create a calming and nurturing environment at home by decluttering, incorporating soothing elements such as soft lighting, comfortable furnishings, and relaxing music or nature sounds.

Reduce Exposure to Toxins: Minimize exposure to environmental toxins and harmful chemicals that may affect reproductive health. Choose organic and natural products whenever possible, and avoid smoking, excessive alcohol consumption, and exposure to pollutants.

Prioritize Sleep: Prioritize quality sleep by establishing a regular sleep schedule, creating a comfortable sleep environment, and practicing good sleep hygiene habits. Aim for 7-9 hours of restful sleep each night to support overall health and fertility.

Stay Informed and Advocacy: Stay informed about your fertility treatment options, rights, and resources available to you. Advocate for yourself and actively participate in decisions regarding your fertility care, ensuring that your voice is heard and your preferences are respected.

By incorporating these strategies into your life, you can create a supportive environment that nurtures your physical, emotional, and mental well-being throughout your fertility journey. Remember that everyone's journey is unique, and it's essential to find what works best for you and seek support when needed.

<u>Please don't forget to rate this book</u>

Thank you

www.ingramcontent.com/pod-product-compliance
Lightning Source LLC
Chambersburg PA
CBHW050905260726
48660CB00001B/29